EKG ECG INTERPRETATION FOR BEGINNERS 2023

A Complete Step-by-Step Guide for Students to Easily Ace Their Exam

By
Martin Thorley

© Copyright 2023 - **All rights reserved - By Martin Thorley**

The content within this book may not be reproduced, duplicated, or transmitted without direct written permission from the author or the publisher.

The information provided herein is stated to be truthful and consistent, in that any liability, in terms of inattention or otherwise, by any usage or abuse of any policies, processes, or directions contained within is the solitary and utter responsibility of the recipient reader. Under no circumstances will any legal responsibility or blame be held against the publisher for any reparation, damages, or monetary loss due to the information herein, either directly or indirectly.

The information herein is offered for informational purposes solely.

This book is not intended to be a substitute for the medical advice of a licensed physician. The reader should consult with their doctor in any matters relating to his/her health.

The presentation of the information is without contract or any type of guarantee assurance.

Readers acknowledge that the author is not engaging in the rendering of legal, financial, medical, or professional advice.

This book is copyright protected.

Table of contents

INTRODUCTION: EKG BASICS 7
- *What is an electrocardiogram (ecg)?* 9
- *History of the ecg* 11
- *How the heart works* 13
- *Ionic and cellular basis of ecg components* 17
- *Importance of ecg interpretation* 19
- *Overview of ecg waves and intervals* 20

CHAPTER 1. ECG LEADS 23
- *Overview of ecg leads* 24
- *Lead placement and positioning* 29
- *Importance of lead placement* 30
- *Electrode types and placement* 31

CHAPTER 2. ECG COMPLEX, WAVES AND INTERVALS . 34
- *Understanding the normal and abnormal p waves of the ecg* 35
- *What are the main deflections on an electrocardiogram?* 36
- *St segment elevation and depression* 38
- *What are the abnormalities of the t wave on an ecg?* 40

CHAPTER 3. ECG RHYTHM ANALYSIS 44
- *Bradycardia* 46
- *What is tachycardia?* 48
- *What is atrial fibrillation?* 50

CHAPTER 4. ECG ISCHEMIA AND INFARCTION............52
ECG ISCHEMIA AND INFARCTION *53*
ISCHEMIA AND INFARCTION..*55*
ECG DIFFERENTIAL DIAGNOSIS OF ISCHEMIA AND INFARCTION.....................*57*
MANAGEMENT OF ECG ISCHEMIA AND INFARCTION.......................................*59*

CHAPTER 5. ECG ARRHYTHMIAS......................................62
OVERVIEW OF ECG ARRHYTHMIAS *64*
TYPES OF ECG ARRHYTHMIAS..*65*
ELECTROCARDIOGRAM FINDINGS IN ARRHYTHMIAS *67*
MANAGEMENT OF ECG ARRHYTHMIAS *69*

CHAPTER 6. ECG MYOCARDIAL ISCHEMIA 71
WHAT ARE THE SIGNS AND SYMPTOMS OF ISCHEMIA?................................*73*
HOW DO YOU FIX MYOCARDIAL ISCHEMIA? *75*
THE DIFFERENCE BETWEEN HEART ATTACK AND ISCHEMIA *76*
WHAT ARE ECG TOOLS?..*78*

CHAPTER 7. EMERGENCY SITUATIONS 81
OVERVIEW OF ECG IN EMERGENCY SITUATIONS..*82*
ECG IN CARDIAC ARREST..*84*
ECG IN SHOCK *86*
ECG IN ACUTE CORONARY SYNDROME..*88*
ST-SEGMENT ELEVATION VERSUS ST-SEGMENT DEPRESSION
ON THE ECG IN ACUTE CORONARY SYNDROME *88*
ELECTROCARDIOGRAM (ECG) IN CARDIOGENIC SHOCK...............................*90*

CHAPTER 8. ECG ARTIFACTS 93
AN OVERVIEW OF ECG ARTIFACTS *94*
TYPES OF ECG ARTIFACTS..*96*
CAUSES OF ECG ARTIFACTS..*98*
ECG ARTIFACT RECOGNITION *101*

CHAPTER 9. ECG INTERPRETATION 103

*REFLECTION ON THE IMPORTANCE OF ECG INTERPRETATION
IN HEALTHCARE 104*

CONCLUSION 107

Introduction: Ekg Basics

The ECG is a graphic representation of cardiac electrical activity displayed on specialized paper that records at a speed of 25mm/second. The height or amplitude of the waveforms reflects differences in voltage across the heart while the width reflects intervals of time.

The first step in reading an ECG is to identify the structure or components that make up the tracing. Each of these components has their definitions, so understanding them will help you quickly recognize deviations from normal.

Waves

The simplest component of the ECG is the wave, which consists of one or more depolarizing waves that travel through the myocardium at a specific rate. The amplitude of the wave is measured in millivolts and the duration in seconds.

Intervals and Segments

The second component of the ECG is an interval, which consists of several waves that move through the heart at different rates. The interval can be broken down into smaller periods called segments. The duration of an interval is also measured in seconds.

QRS Complexes

The third component of the ECG is the QRS complex, which

consists of the QRS and P waves. The QRS complex is generally the largest wave on the ECG, so it is important to quickly determine its duration.

PR Interval

The PR interval varies slightly from patient to patient depending on the rate of excitation. This is usually between 0.2 and 0.04 seconds.

Large Squares

The large squares that appear between the QRS waves are an indication of the depolarization rate of the ventricles. It takes approximately 30 large squares for the ventricles to depolarize.

A small square between the R waves and the next QRS complex indicates a slower rate of depolarization. This may indicate a pacemaker or sinus node failure.

Direction of Waveforms

The direction of depolarizing waves is important in interpreting the ECG. This is done by using a concept known as vector theory.

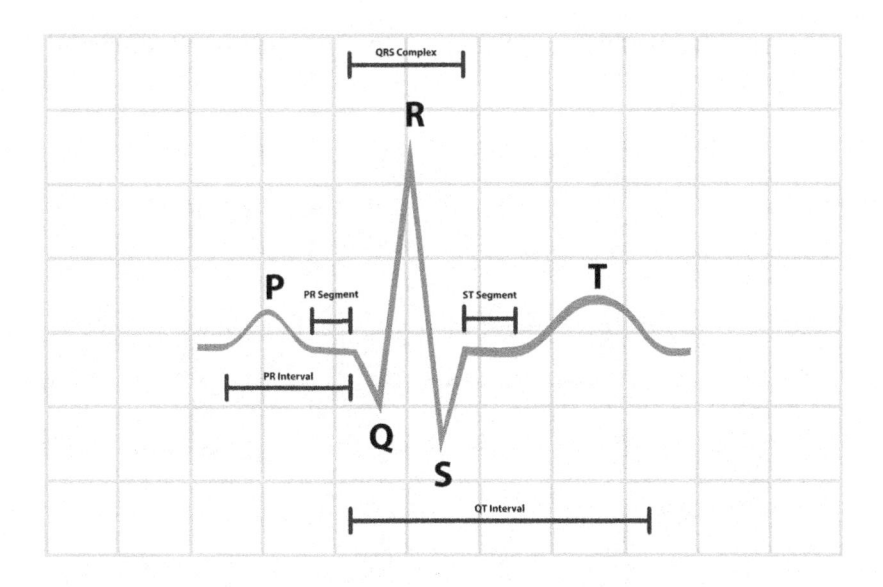

Lead Polarity and the Direction of Waveforms

The polarity of each of the ECG's lead is determined by which electrodes on the patient's body are connected to the heart. If one or more of the limb leads is incorrectly connected, the result will be an abnormal lead pattern.

What is an Electrocardiogram (ECG)?

An electrocardiogram (ECG) is a test that can help to detect problems with your heart, such as a heart rhythm problem. It's often carried out by a doctor who specializes in heart health. ECG tests can reveal a wide range of heart conditions, including a fluttering or irregular heart rhythm, abnormal heart activity, a heart valve problem, coronary artery disease or an enlarged heart.

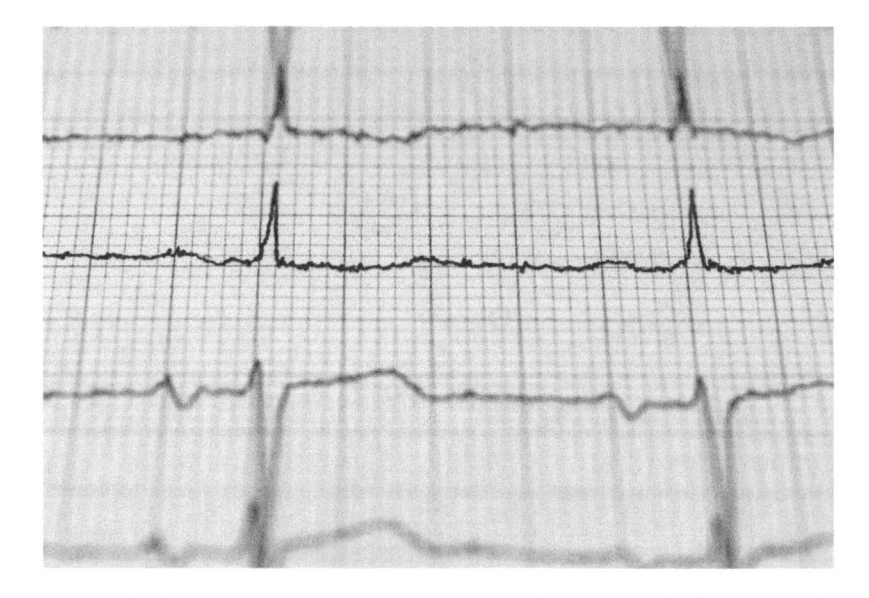

When the electrodes are in place, they pick up electrical signals from your heart that are sent by your muscles as they contract to pump blood around the body. The machine that records the ECG converts these signals into a series of wavy lines called "waves" and saves them on paper or in a computer file.

If you're having an exercise stress test, the electrodes are put on while you do exercises - such as riding a bike or walking on a treadmill. They are removed once the test is over.

The electrodes are connected to a recording device that lets the doctor see all the wavy lines of an ECG at once, as well as the individual waves that make up each one. Each individual wave tells the doctor what part of the heart is active. This can help to spot areas that might be struggling under physical stress and give your doctor an idea of how well your heart is working overall.

A number of special features are used to protect the ECG from dangerous situations, such as electrostatic discharge and defibrillation. These include low noise circuitry, instrumentation amplifiers and electromagnetic shielding to reduce common-mode interference.

It's also a good idea to tell your doctor if you have any unusual symptoms after an ECG, such as chest pain, shortness of breath or dizziness. You'll be asked to change into a hospital gown and remove any jewellery or other items that might interfere with the ECG. You'll also need to lie down on an examining table or bed. It's important to stay still and not talk during the test, so that the tracing isn't altered.

History of the ECG

The ECG (Electrocardiogram) is a test that measures the small electric waves that the heart creates. It has been a mainstay of medical technology for over a century and is used worldwide to diagnose heart disease, including coronary artery disease.

The history of electrocardiography dates back to the late 1700s when James Mackenzie, in Aberdeen, Scotland, first began studying the pulse with the use of a home-made polygraph. He subsequently introduced a number of innovations in electrocardiography such as the use of pails of conducting solution for recording ECG leads and the concept of using a galvanometer to measure electrical impulses.

In 1872, Gabriel Lippman in New York came up with a capillary electrometer that could be used to measure voltages on the skin. He also pioneered the use of two-wire electrodes that allowed the ECG to be recorded from multiple electrodes simultaneously.

A decade later, Willem Einthoven developed a galvanometer that could be used to measure the amplitudes of electrical currents generated by the heart and was awarded the Nobel Prize in Medicine in 1924. This galvanometer, which weighed 600 pounds and took five people to operate, was the forerunner of many later advances in ECG technology.

From this time on, electrocardiography was a major area of research and development by scientists in Europe, the US and elsewhere. By the late 1950s, a number of attempts to automate the interpretation of ECGs had begun and this work had gained momentum. The first such program was based on three simultaneous orthogonal leads and commenced in 1957 at the Veteran's Administration Hospital in Washington DC, under the direction of Dr. Hubert V. Pip Berger.

This technique was successful and was subsequently replicated by a variety of different manufacturers. The advent of a standard format for data transmission between manufacturers' equipment - known as the Standard Communications Protocol (SCP) - was a major contribution to this development, enabling ECG data from different vendors' machines to be interpreted in a common way. This was particularly helpful in facilitating comparisons between ECGs from different sources, such as between hospital systems and commercially available electrocardiographs.

How the Heart Works

The heart is a muscle responsible for pumping blood throughout the body. The ECG records these electrical impulses, allowing physicians to diagnose heart conditions and monitor the heart's electrical activity. Over the years, the technology of ECG machines has greatly improved, becoming smaller, more portable, and easier to use. Today, ECGs are commonly used in a variety of medical settings, including hospitals, clinics, and even in the home. In addition to the standard 12-lead ECG, there are also more advanced forms of ECG such as Holter monitors, which allow for continuous monitoring of the heart's electrical activity over a period of time, and event monitors, which are used to record ECG data during symptoms or when the patient activates the device.

The ECG has proven to be a crucial diagnostic tool in the evaluation of heart conditions, including arrhythmias, heart attacks, and certain heart diseases. ECG results can help healthcare providers determine the presence and severity of heart problems, and assist in developing appropriate treatment plans the healthcare provider will interpret the EKG to determine if the heart is functioning normally and if there are any heart rhythm problems. It's important to note that an EKG is just one of many tests used to evaluate heart health, and it may not provide a complete picture of a person's heart health.

In conclusion, the ECG is an important tool for understanding the electrical activity of the heart and diagnosing heart conditions. Its development and improvement over the years has greatly contributed to our understanding of the heart and improved patient care.

Blood Flow of the Human Heart

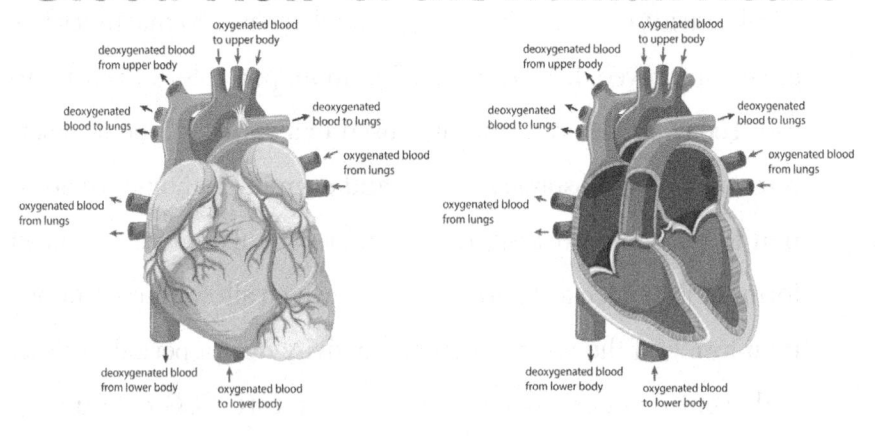

The heart is made up of multiple layers of tissue and a complex network of vessels. The heart pumps blood around the body, providing oxygen and nutrients to organs and removing carbon dioxide and wastes.

A normal healthy heart pumps about 2,000 gallons of blood each day. This works hard to keep the rest of the body going, so it is important for you to understand how the heart works.

Your heart has four chambers that divide the body into left and right sides. These are called the atria and ventricles, and each has its own valve.

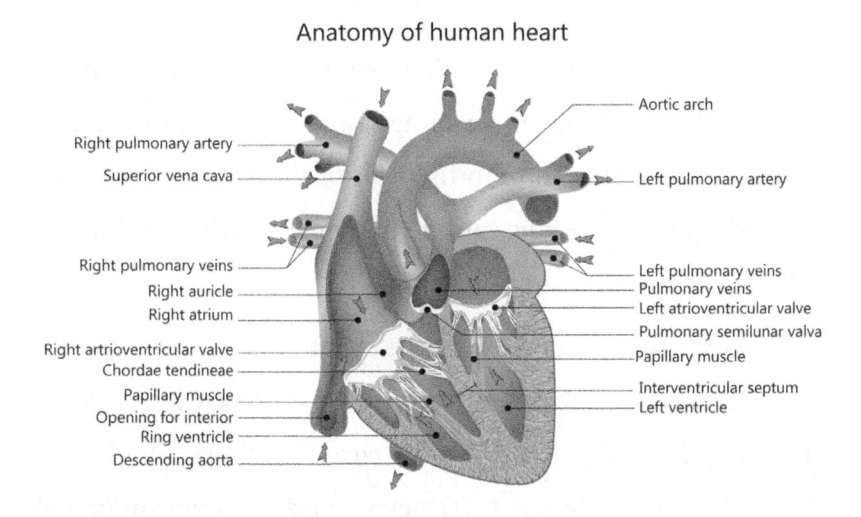

Anatomy of human heart

- Aortic arch
- Right pulmonary artery
- Superior vena cava
- Left pulmonary artery
- Right pulmonary veins
- Right auricle
- Right atrium
- Left pulmonary veins
- Pulmonary veins
- Left atrioventricular valve
- Pulmonary semilunar valva
- Right artrioventricular valve
- Chordae tendineae
- Papillary muscle
- Papillary muscle
- Opening for interior
- Ring ventricle
- Interventricular septum
- Left ventricle
- Descending aorta

At rest, your heart may beat 60 to 100 times a minute (bpm). But it can rise to 100 bpm or more during exercise. The heart's rate is regulated by a special cluster of cells in the right atrium, called the sinus node. The sinus node prompts the upper chambers to contract first and then sends an electrical impulse to a second cluster of cells between the upper and lower chambers, which triggers the ventricles to contract.

When the upper chambers of your heart contract, the blood from the right atrium flows to your right ventricle. The lungs use the oxygen in your blood to help you breathe and remove the carbon dioxide.

Once the blood is in the lungs, it enters tiny capillaries on the surface of the lungs' air sacs. This process supplies oxygen and removes carbon dioxide from the blood, enabling it to travel from your lungs through the arteries to the heart.

After entering the lungs, the blood enters your coronary arteries (branches of the aorta). The right and left coronary arteries supply oxygen-rich blood to the wall of the myocardium. The myocardium is a working muscle that needs oxygen and nutrients to contract efficiently.

This nutrient-rich blood then passes into a system of cardiac veins and leaves your heart through the coronary sinus. Most of the cardiac veins drain into the coronary sinus, which then opens into your right atrium. Once you have a large volume of deoxygenated blood in the right atrium, it is drained through your pulmonic valve.

Your lungs need oxygen to function properly, but most of the blood in your body is oxygen-poor. This blood returns to the heart through two main veins, called the superior and inferior vena cava.

The superior vena cava and the inferior vena cava empty oxygen-poor blood into the right atrium.

The aorta is the largest artery in the body, which takes blood from your heart and branches into many smaller arteries that distribute oxygenated blood to organs throughout the body. The aorta also connects to the heart to pick up oxygenated blood from the left ventricle. This circulatory blood flow is the basis for all systemic circulation.

Ionic and Cellular Basis of ECG Components

The ECG is a record of the electrical activity of the heart in real time. The basic waveforms of an ECG tracing are called J (Osborn) waves, ST-segment displacement, T-wave and U-wave. They dynamically change in morphology under various pathophysiologic conditions and play an important role in the development of ventricular arrhythmias.

Classification of ECGs:

1) abnormal variants of what is considered normal

2) abnormal findings that are less common and may represent an arrhythmia or other serious condition. It is therefore essential to know the basic properties of these waves, how they are produced and how to recognize them in an ECG.

a. J-Wave, ST-Segment Displacement and T-Wave

The genesis of the J (Osborn) wave on the ECG is associated with electrical heterogeneity between ventricular epicardium, M cells, and endocardium during ventricular repolarization. The underlying mechanism involves the difference in transmural voltage gradient due to differences in the Ito-mediated AP notch between the ventricular epicardium and endocardium. The exaggeration of this gradient in certain pathologic states has been linked to the development of polymorphic ventricular tachycardias, such as torsade de pointes.

b. ST-Segment Displacement, Elevation and Depression

The appearance of ST segment depressions in the anterior leads is similar to that of physical exercise or hy-perventilation.

QTc Interval Conclusion: The QT interval is the shortest period between the end of the QRS complex and its beginning. It is measured in milliseconds and is calculated automatically on most modern ECG machines.

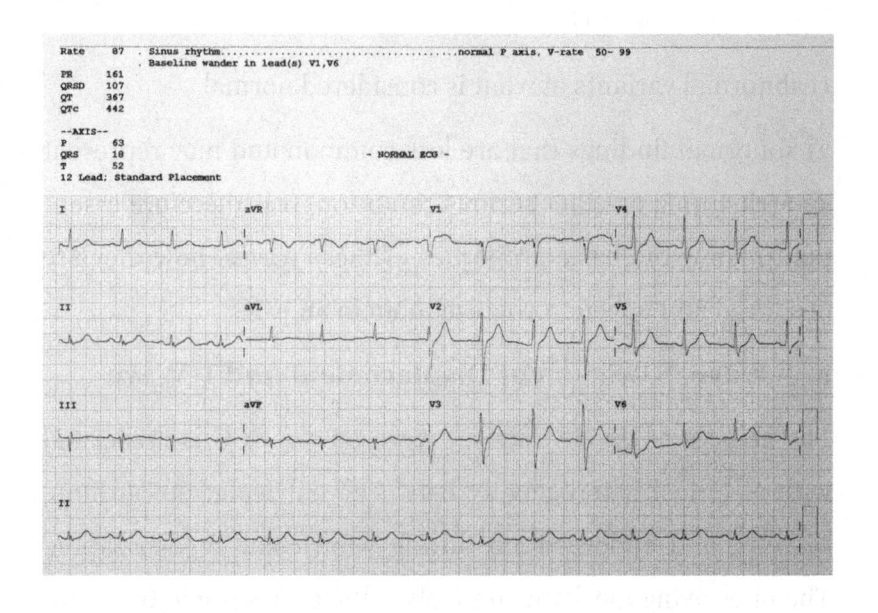

Importance of ECG Interpretation

It is also used to diagnose and monitor heart disease, and to screen for conditions that can affect the electrolytes in the bloodstream, such as hypokalemia or hypocalcemia. It is especially helpful for identifying abnormalities of the ventricular conduction system or cardiac arrhythmias.

In clinical practice, a number of recommendations for the standardization and interpretation of ECGs have been made over the years. These have been endorsed by the American Heart Association (AHA and are essential for effective patient care. These include the development of a single, comprehensive lexicon of descriptive, diagnostic and modifying terminology for the ECG; standardization of recording techniques and lead placements; use of computerized ECG instruments to improve efficiency; and quality assurance.

However, many medical professionals do not fully understand the importance of ECG interpretation. This is a concern because ECG interpretation is an essential part of healthcare that requires knowledge and skill.

There are many ways to gain ECG knowledge and skills, including reading textbooks or practicing with ECG cases. Whether you are an aspiring nurse or a current nurse professional, it is important to learn about the different ECG waves, segments and intervals that can be found on a typical 12-lead EKG.

This will ensure that you know how to interpret an ECG and how to determine if it is normal or not.

In addition, it is important to pay attention to lead placement as this will have an impact on your ability to interpret the ECG correctly. If you notice a pattern of tachycardia, for example, and the leads do not appear to be on properly, or are not positioned correctly, it can significantly influence your interpretation. If you see a rapid, irregular rhythm that looks like it could be putting your patient into a lethal heart rhythm, you should consider referring them to a specialist.

Despite the importance of ECG interpretation, many medical students and young doctors feel that their skills in ECG interpretation are not up to par. This has prompted research into new methods to teach these skills.

Overview of ECG Waves and Intervals

Waves (positive and negative deflections from baseline) are grouped together to form a complex, which is the main component of an ECG. Each wave can be classified as a specific type of electrical event. For example, the P wave represents a change in the electrical potential across the left and right atria. This pause allows blood to flow into the ventricles before contraction and ejection can occur.

The QRS complex is an important part of the ECG because it reflects the ventricular depolarization process (upstrokes and downstrokes). It is the shortest segment on the ECG and is less than 0.12 seconds in duration.

QRS Complex - The most important wave on an ECG, the QRS complex is a series of 3 deflections that represent ventricular depolarization. It is usually less than 0.12 seconds in duration and consists of 3'small squares', each one being 1 mm in height.

U Wave - Not visible on a normal ECG, the U wave indicates repolarization of the Purkinje fibers. It is a very small wave and is usually located after the T wave on an ECG.

T Wave - Inverted in every lead except aVR, the T wave identifies ventricular depolarization and indicates the ventricles are relaxing. It may also represent ischemia, especially if it is combined with LVH and ST depression.

Long QT Interval - A prolonged or abnormally long period of depolarization and repolarization on an ECG (QT interval). It can indicate conditions that prolong the heart's ability to beat, such as cardiac arrhythmias and hypertension.

This is a very important section of an ECG that is often overlooked because it can be difficult to read. It is important to remember that each ECG is unique and should be interpreted in conjunction with the rate, rhythm and axis. An ECG must be systematically analyzed and reviewed to avoid missing anything. This means that you should always start by looking at the rate, rhythm and axis and then move to the waves, segments and intervals. This is an excellent technique for interpreting

ECGs and will help you to quickly catch any problems that could be present.

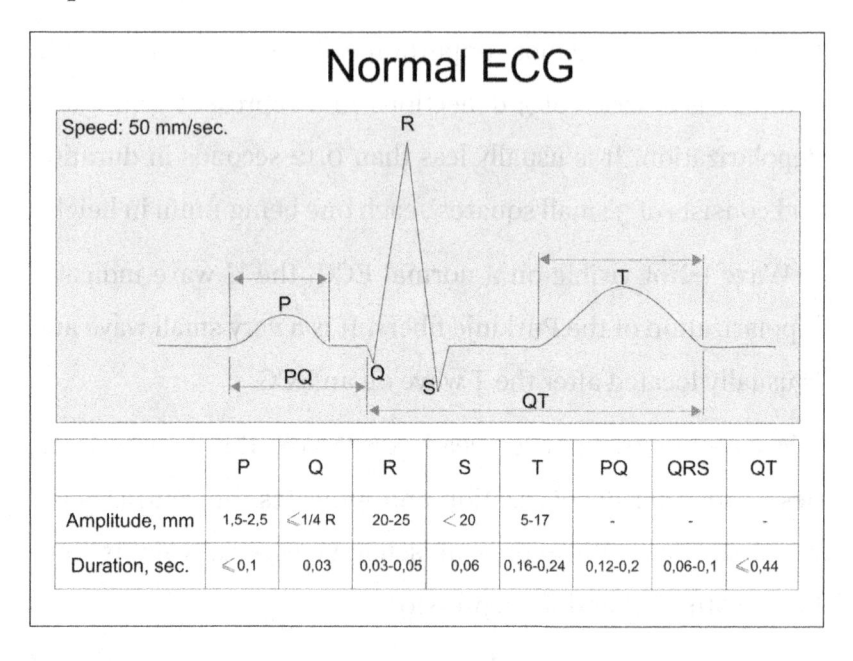

Normal ECG

Speed: 50 mm/sec.

	P	Q	R	S	T	PQ	QRS	QT
Amplitude, mm	1,5-2,5	≤1/4 R	20-25	<20	5-17	-	-	-
Duration, sec.	≤0,1	0,03	0,03-0,05	0,06	0,16-0,24	0,12-0,2	0,06-0,1	≤0,44

Chapter 1.
ECG Leads

ECG leads are a graphical representation of electrical activity generated by the heart's atria and ventricles. They are computed from the data recorded by various electrodes attached to the patient's skin. The tracings are used to diagnose a variety of conditions, including arrhythmias and morphological changes (e.g., ischemia and infarction).

The 12-lead system of ECGs comprises a total of 12 "electrical positions" on the heart that give a three-dimensional view of the heart's electrical activity from different angles. Each lead is designed to pick up a specific "position" of the electrical currents within the heart, providing a more accurate diagnosis than that obtained by one single view.

The placement of the leads varies from patient to patient, as does their location relative to the nipples. For male patients, the electrodes are usually placed on the right arm and left upper arm, while for female patients they are typically placed under the left breast.

All leads in the 12-lead system have a reference point, and are therefore bipolar (positive/negative). The difference in voltage between the exploring electrode and the reference point yields a wave or deflection. The vector - which is the direction of the movement of the wave - is represented by an arrow, and this is the basis for interpreting ECG tracings.

Ideally, each lead should be placed directly on dry skin, avoiding the use of any lotions or oils that may interfere with its reading. Electrodes should also be carefully sterilized, as expired ones can cause confusion in the interpretation of a tracing.

Some manufacturers of electrodes stress that they should be shaved when necessary, and should be removed from air tight packages to avoid any contamination. They also recommend that the electrodes be placed on the skin with a minimum of dead skin cells as these can affect the ECG results.

These modified systems, which can be found in most cardiac monitors, generate ECG tracings with amplitudes and durations that differ from the conventional 12-lead system. They can be used to detect a wide range of cardiac conditions, including arrhythmias, but are not recommended for detecting morphological conditions because the alternative electrode placement may alter criteria that depend on amplitude and interval.

Overview of ECG leads

A standard 12-lead ECG records a complete tracing of the heart's electrical activity from 12 different "electrical positions" on the heart muscle. The standard ECG is made up of 6 chest leads and 3 limb leads (the left leg and the arms). Each of these three limbs leads acts like a wire connecting to one of three points on the torso – known as Einthoven's triangle – named after Wilhelm Einthoven who invented the first practical ECG machine.

Right-sided and left-sided leads are made up of six limb leads, with V4R and V6R placed on the right side of the body, and leads V7-V8-V9 placed on the left. These lead systems allow for the detection of a number of abnormalities that would otherwise be inaccessible with traditional ECGs, including right ventricular infarction and ischemia.

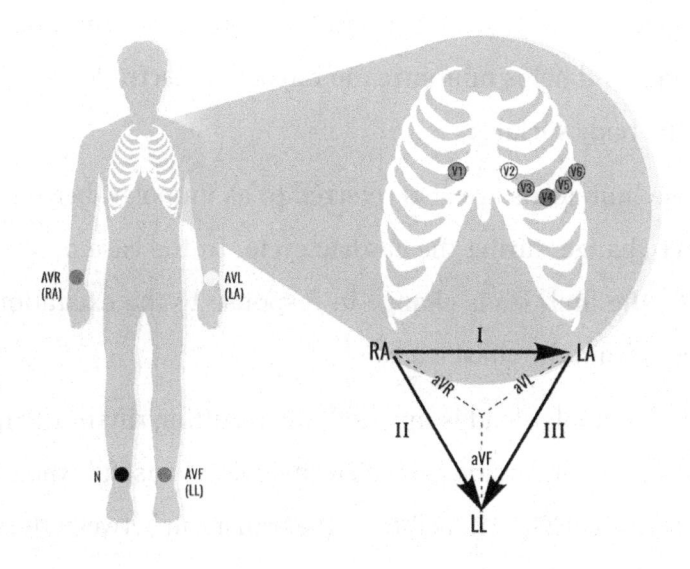

Limb leads comprise the four electrodes that are placed on each limb. They are connected to the ECG recorder via a cable, which measures the potential difference between these electrodes in millivolts.

Each of these six limb leads is angled slightly differently in relation to the frontal plane, which affects how they detect vectors from this plane. Hence, they produce ECG waves with varying amplitudes and axes as a result.

As a rule of thumb, it is recommended that the left and right arm electrodes are in the same plane as the chest leads. This allows for the best possible accuracy in diagnosing cardiac ischemia and detecting left ventricular infarction.

In addition to the left and right arm leads, each limb also has a lead that is considered a neutral lead, similar to an electric plug. This is used to provide a grounding point that minimizes ECG artifact and helps minimize the impact of electrodes that aren't on the body surface.

These limb leads are also referred to as unipolar, because they don't change during the cardiac cycle. In the case of a bipolar ECG, the limb leads change in response to the excitation that occurs from the chest leads.

When a bipolar lead is inverted, the resulting rhythm strip also has an aVR inversion. The aVR inversion is useful when interpreting an ECG, as it facilitates the transition between the waveforms in neighboring leads.

Electrocardiography is a noninvasive way of observing the electrical activity of the heart. The electrical currents that occur inside the heart are recorded by electrodes attached to the skin and analyzed by an ECG monitor. The resulting graphic description of the heart's electrical activity is called an electrocardiogram (ECG).

Type of ECG Leads

There are a number of different types of ECG leads, each designed to analyze specific events and record them in a more accurate manner than others. The limb leads measure a 360-degree copulate circle around the heart that includes 306 degrees of the frontal plane axis. This gives them the ability to observe all of the cardiac electrical activity from all possible angles, making them very sensitive to any conduction deft in the heart.

In addition, these limb leads are angled at a variety of angles that will detect the vectors traveling through different frontal and horizontal planes. This information is useful in determining the presence of various pathological changes such as arrhythmias, cardiomyopathy and cardiac tumors.

Common Lead Placement Errors

A major source of confusion and misunderstanding when performing ECGs is the placement of the ECG leads. This can result in errors that can create artifacts, mimic pathological findings or even interfere with proper ECG interpretation.

Lead placement is a very important aspect of the performance of electrocardiography and can make or break a patient's health. A good lead position is essential for the accurate and reliable diagnosis of cardiac conditions such as arrhythmias, ventricular hypertrophy and heart failure.

The ECG trace quality depends on a number of factors including the skin's resistance, the position of the electrodes, the temperature of the patient and the amount of time the electrodes are in contact with the skin. The best tracings are obtained when the electrodes are fully in contact with the skin, which is achieved by using dry, non-alcohol wipes that have been wiped with a soapy solution or water.

Another factor influencing the tracing quality is the location of the electrodes, which should be placed in a central position that will record both P- and QRS waves. This placement will allow the tracing to reflect the ventricular activation cycle and provide the most accurate picture of the heart's electrical activity.

An additional factor that can influence the tracing quality is the electrodes' polarity, which is important for interpreting ECGs. A negative lead will not display the repolarization waveform and may have a flat amplitude, while a positive lead will show a peak or inverted T-wave.

Other factors that affect the tracing quality are the size and shape of the electrodes, which can change their resistance to electricity, as well as the thickness and properties of the intervening tissues. For example, a large electrode that is not in close contact with the myocardium will increase the amount of voltage required to generate an ECG waveform, and can cause the T-wave to be either inverted or elevated.

Lead placement and positioning

When a patient has an ECG, it's important that the electrodes are placed in a way that will yield correct waveforms. Misplaced leads can result in incorrect readings and may contribute to misdiagnosis. Moreover, errors in lead placement can disrupt stratification and management efforts for patients with cardiac disease.

The ECG can provide information about the heart's electrical activity from a variety of angles, including vertical and horizontal planes. There are 10 electrodes in a 12-lead ECG that give 12 different perspectives, or views of the heart's activity. Each view provides information about vectors in that plane, which are the paths that cardiac impulses travel through the heart.

How do I position the chest leads?

When placing chest leads, it is helpful to use bone landmarks for correct positioning.

It is also important to locate the fourth intercostal space (ICS) for accurate chest lead placement. This is the junction between the clavicle and sternum, which can be located by palpating the upper sternum or by sliding your fingers down the center of the sternum until you feel a bony prominence.

Next, place the chest leads on a vertical or horizontal plane on the body. When a lead is placed on the head, it will primarily record vectors traveling in the frontal plane; when a lead is placed on the sternum, it will primarily record vectors traveling from the sternum to the anterior chest wall.

Once the lead has been positioned, it will be snared by a guidewire and advanced to the coronary sinus (CS) through a venous access point, usually at the back of the chest, using a snaring procedure. If a CS is not accessible, the electrode can be placed in the torso or on the femoral artery.

The torso is a difficult place to place the chest leads, as a torso is a relatively large structure that makes it difficult to get an optimal view of the CS vasculature. Additionally, the torso can often be twisted or bent during an ECG session. As such, torso lead positioning can be an unsettling experience for both the ECG technician and the patient, leading to inaccurate interpretations.

Importance of lead placement

Having the right leads in the right places can make a huge difference when it comes to assessing and managing patients with cardiac conditions. Not only can misplaced electrodes be confusing for patients and providers alike, they can also cause a host of recording issues.

In particular, errors involving electrode placement have been linked to a number of sex related inequities that can impact patient outcomes. This is particularly true of women, who are known to be more likely to experience physiological differences that can influence their ECG responses.

Leads and their occupants

To get the best possible results, ECG professionals should consider the nuances of their patients' anatomy, physiology, and preferences. While this may require a bit of sleuthing, the result will be more accurate readings that will lead to more informed care and a happier, healthier patient.

In short, the correct placement of all of your 12 leads is a crucial part of delivering optimal diagnostics in a timely fashion. The best way to do this is to incorporate the following tips and tricks into your daily practice.

Electrode types and placement

They determine the range of voltages and currents that may be recorded by an e. electrode, and they can affect the amount of muscle activation that can be recorded.

The most common electrode types are those that are based on the limb leads (I, II, III, aVF, aVR and aVL) or on the chest (V1, V2, V3, V4, V5, and V6). The limb and chest leads have the exploring electrodes and reference points located in frontal and horizontal planes, respectively, so that they can detect vectors that travel in these planes.

ECG

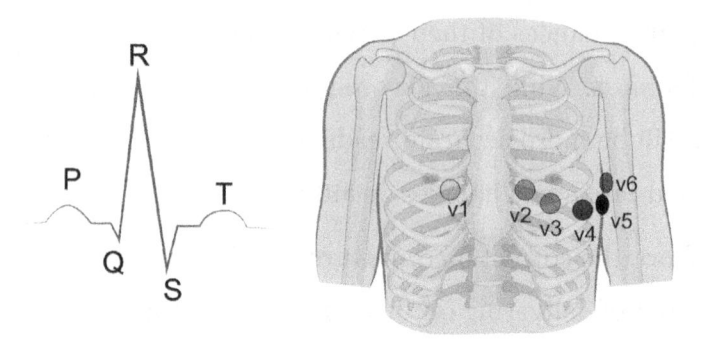

However, there are some problems associated with conventional limb and chest electrode placement, which can prevent the recording of optimal EEGs in various clinical situations. When a patient is receiving electrical nerve stimulation for the treatment of Parkinson's disease, it is important to choose an electrode configuration that will result in the best EEG results. This can be achieved by considering the distance between the electrodes and the hippocampi in order to determine the best placement.

Self-adhesive and carbon-impregnated electrodes were used in a crossover design that allowed comparison of the effects of electrode type and configuration on all outcome measures. Despite the fact that BT placement has a higher hippocampal ROI EF than RUL or BF placements, the difference is not statistically significant. This is probably because the BT placement has a longer distance between the electrodes and the hippocampi, which may increase shunting of current from the electrode to the brain due to electrical resistance in the skull. This decreases EF in the dAC ROI and results in a lower EF overall. The BF placement is a more traditional placement that has been used in the past and results in lower EF in the dAC ROI than both BT and RUL. This is likely due to a longer distance between the electrodes and a smaller hippocampal volume, which may allow more current to penetrate to the brain.

Chapter 2.
ECG Complex, Waves and Intervals

It reveals a picture of normal heart function and is an invaluable diagnostic tool in detecting and treating cardiac abnormalities. Using the ECG to diagnose cardiology-related problems is the key to successful patient care and outcomes.

The atrial atrioventricular node, also known as the AV node, is a compact area of conducting tissue near the coronary sinus. This node is responsible for connecting impulses from the atria to the ventricular bundle branches, which comprise rapidly conducting fibers called Purkinje fibers.

QRS Complex– The largest spike on the ECG corresponding to ventricular depolarization represents the start of systole and ventricle contraction. This phase of the cardiac cycle lasts approximately 270 ms.

R wave– The next smallest wave on the ECG corresponding with ventricular depolarization represents the start of the R-wave, the most important phase of systole, and the beginning of the ventricles' contraction. The R-wave represents the peak of the QRS complex. Large amplitudes of the R and S waves represent left ventricular hypertrophy.

T wave– The largest wave on the ECG corresponding with repolarization of the ventricles demonstrates the refractory period of contractile cells and indicates the end of the systole.

Understanding the Normal and Abnormal P Waves of the ECG

Abnormal P waves are associated with pathologic conditions such as atrial fibrillation, arrhythmogenic right ventricular dysfunction, valvular heart diseases, rheumatologic disorders, idiopathic hypertension, and congenital heart defects.

These abnormalities are often observed in a variety of different clinical settings and can provide information regarding the presence, severity, and course of disease, as well as the ability to predict the occurrence of AF or a heart block if one exists.

P wave duration is a useful measure of diastolic dysfunction. In patients with AF, prolonged P waves have been shown to be associated with increased office systolic blood pressure (BP) and higher heart rates on echocardiography. In addition, increased P-wave duration is associated with left atrial (LA) dilatation and LVH, which have been shown to be predictive of future cardiac events.

However, despite these findings, there are still many questions regarding the clinical relevance of these findings and whether or not a patient's risk of cardiac events is directly related to P-wave duration. In fact, a recent study in Japanese outpatients with CV risks demonstrated that a P-wave width of > 140 ms is a better predictor of cardiovascular events than a P-wave duration of more than 120 ms [9].

In contrast, studies have shown that a longer P-wave duration is not a reliable indicator of cardiac events in individuals without CV risk factors and may have limited usefulness for those with these factors.

A high degree of sensitivity and specificity has been shown for the assessment of P-wave duration in different clinical situations, such as the diagnosis of atrial fibrillation in patients with no apparent heart disease, in hypertensive individuals, in a wide range of coronary artery disease patients and in a variety of congenital and rheumatologic diseases. In the clinical setting, a spline-like model with a smoothing amplitude of 80 to 180 milliseconds has been used to evaluate the association between P-wave duration and AF. Among AF cases, a higher proportion of cases with abnormal morphology were associated with AF than those without abnormal morphology. This finding was not observed in controls. This was particularly true for cases with advanced interatrial blocks (IAB) and for those with partial IAB.

What Are the Main Deflections on an Electrocardiogram?

In a standard ECG, the main deflections are the QRS complex (R and S) and the T wave. The Q wave represents the ventricular depolarization and the S wave represents the repolarization of the ventricles.

When the ventricular muscles are not functioning properly, a wide and/or long QRS complex indicates that there is a problem in the conduction system. These conditions may be associated with cardiac arrhythmias or sudden death.

Large amplitudes of the QRS complex also indicate left ventricular hypertrophy or enlargement. This is because the electrical currents generated by the ventricular myocardium are proportional to the ventricular muscle mass.

This is because the ventricular muscle cells are closer together than those in an obese individual. A slender person may also have smaller and less dilated coronary arteries that supply blood to the heart.

Slender individuals may also have decreased ventricular contractility and this causes the QRS complex to be short. This is due to the fact that the ventricular myocardium may not generate enough energy for sufficient impulses to reach the electrodes.

When the ventricular myocardium is working normally, the amplitude of the QRS complex is usually 80 to 120 ms. However, this varies with different ECG recording leads and in people with abnormal conduction within the ventricles.

In addition to the QRS complex, there are other deflections on an ECG that can be useful in assessing electrical activity in the heart. It must not be too long or too short and a normal PR interval varies between 0.12 seconds and 0.22 seconds.

Another feature of the QRS complex that is of importance to medical doctors is the J point. The ST segment is an isoelectric region of the ECG that occurs after the QRS complex.

ST Segment Elevation and Depression

ST segment elevation (STE) or depression is a feature of electrocardiograms that indicates myocardial injury. It represents a change in the electrical properties of a cardiac muscle, which is caused by inflammation or an abnormality in contractile function. It is a characteristic of acute myocardial infarction and is associated with a risk of necrosis. It is a common feature of ischemic heart disease, but there are many non-cardiac diseases that can also cause ST elevation and ST depression on an ECG.

Acute myocardial ischemia causes a disruption of the myocardium's membrane potential during phase 2 of the heart cycle (ventricular systole). This is the period when the heart contracts and is subject to depolarization from the AV node. The ST segment is displaced upwards, which is known as an ST elevation, or downwards, which is known as an ST depression.

Ischemia-related ST elevations can be straight or convex, depending on the type of ischemia. A straight ST segment is more specific for ischemia than a convex one.

There are several conditions that can mimic myocardial infarction on an ECG, including pulmonary embolism (PE), pneumothorax, and pericarditis. Other conditions include COVID-19, gastrointestinal bleeding, and abdominal aortic aneurysm.

Other non-cardiac diseases that can produce ST-segment elevation on an ECG include hepatitis B, hepatitis C, and chronic liver disease. The most important of these is hepatitis B because it is associated with a disproportionately high rate of myocardial infarction, which can lead to death in patients with acute coronary syndrome.

In addition to hepatitis, other common conditions that can produce ST-segment changes on an ECG include pulmonary embolism, hypertension, hypotension, and cardiogenic shock. These conditions can be challenging to diagnose because the ECG changes are so dynamic and often do not reflect any prior ECG changes.

Symptoms that may be associated with a non-cardiac condition with a ST segment elevation on an ECG include shortness of breath, chest pain, and dizziness. Detection of these symptoms in conjunction with a positive ECG can help to distinguish a patient's condition from that of an acute myocardial infarction.

Non-cardiac ST segment elevations are more likely to occur in a convex shape than an upsloping or horizontal shape. This is because a convex shape is more consistent with an acute myocardial infarction than an upsloping or horizontal shape.

Reciprocal STD is another condition that can appear in leads that are not demonstrating ST elevation. It is more likely to occur in anterior leads and less likely to appear in inferior leads. It is thought that reciprocal change is secondary to a combination of factors including coexisting ischemia, infarct extension, and a displacement of the injury current vector away from the myocardium that is not infected.

Regardless of the cause, the presence of a depressed but upsloping ST segment on an ECG usually rules out ischemia as the underlying cause. However, in certain situations this finding can suggest an underlying condition that requires invasive testing. Ischemic ST depressions generally show a horizontal or downsloping ST segment, which is required by North American and European guidelines.

What Are the Abnormalities of the T Wave on an ECG?

T wave represents the time interval during which ventricular repolarization occurs on the surface electrocardiogram (ECG) during ventricular diastole. They provide valuable clues to underlying pathology and can be used to evaluate cardiovascular risk in patients with various clinical syndromes.

T-wave morphology

The morphology of T waves is a very important part of the diagnostic evaluation of ECGs, as it provides information on the degree of ventricular repolarization and the presence of arrhythmias. T-wave morphology can be correlated with several clinical syndromes including congestive heart failure, low ejection fraction, and acute myocardial infarction. It is also useful for evaluating the response to therapeutic interventions such as drug therapies or exercise stress testing.

Electrocardiography

Normal sinus rhythm

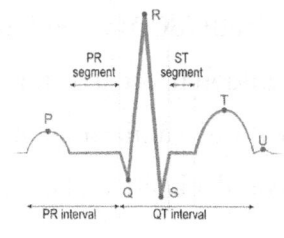

ST Elevated Myocardial Infarction

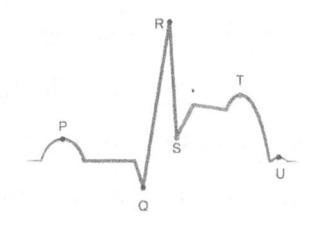

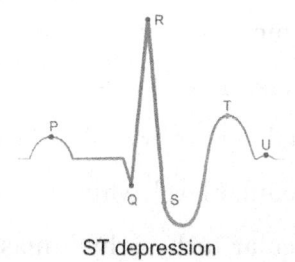

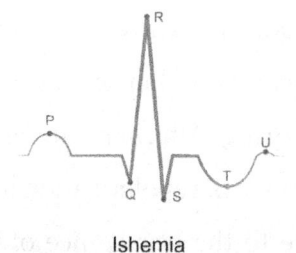

ST depression

Ishemia

Giant negative T waves or GNTs are negatively-oriented T waves with amplitude greater than 10 mm and a peak at 1 mV that occur in the precordial leads. These are commonly seen in patients with coronary artery disease, hypertrophic cardiomyopathy, long QT syndromes (LQTS), and cerebrovascular accidents. In these patients, T-wave morphology is accompanied by a variety of changes in the spatial dispersion of repolarization.

Asymmetrical T waves are often seen in the post-ischemic period after cardiac ischemia and are usually seen in the chest leads, particularly V1-V3. These T-waves are broad in amplitude and can vary in height from -1.0 mm to +1.0 mm. Asymmetrical T waves are often seen in combination with flat T-waves and a small U-wave.

Variable T-wave amplitude and morphology are considered to be a positive diagnostic feature in patients with ventricular tachyarrhythmias or sudden cardiac death (SCD) when they occur in conjunction with a history of sudden heart arrest. During exercise stress testing, a decrease in T-wave amplitude or morphology is associated with an increased likelihood of sudden cardiac arrest.

Alternans of T-wave amplitude and morphology can be detected by means of either exercise stress testing or long-term Holter monitoring. Alternans are associated with every-other-beat alternations of repolarization at the cellular level, which may contribute to the occurrence of ventricular tachyarrhythmias and SCD.

These alterations of repolarization at the cellular and subcellular levels are thought to be critical to the development and pathophysiology of SCD and malignant arrhythmias. However, the exact mechanism by which T-wave amplitude and morphology alter is unclear. Currently, TWA analysis is not used as part of routine clinical practice to evaluate the susceptibility of patients with cardiac disease to lethal arrhythmias.

T-wave inversions are a common feature of ECGs in patients with cardiac disease, especially in elderly patients. T-wave inversions may be symmetric or non-symmetric, and are associated with a number of conditions including acute coronary artery disease, myocardial infarction, and pulmonary embolism.

Acute coronary artery disease is the most common clinical condition associated with T-wave inversions on the ECG. In an elderly population, T-wave inversions are associated with a higher risk of CHD compared to ECGs without T-wave inversions. These findings support the use of T-wave inversions on the ECG in predicting cardiovascular risk.

Chapter 3.
ECG Rhythm Analysis

A good ECG is essential to a cardiologist's arsenal of tools and techniques. It can reveal a patient's heart condition in the blink of an eye.

Besides the stethoscope, the ECG is one of the oldest and most enduring medical devices used by humans. It is a plot of electrical voltage on a vertical axis against time on a horizontal axis.

The ECG is a collection of 10 electrodes (eight to the right and left sides of the body) that record electrical activity in the heart and its blood vessels.

A systematic approach to interpretation of the ECG is vital for a quick and accurate diagnosis in order to save a patient's life. The ECG is an amazing technology that allows us to detect heart disease and treat it before it is too late. The most important step is to learn how to read it and understand the underlying science behind it.

ECG rhythm analysis is a critical skill for nurses and doctors to have. It requires a good theoretical foundation in cardiac arrhythmias, a keen eye and a knowledge of the heart's conduction and the EKG machine itself. A normal heart beats in an organized manner with P waves moving regularly across the strip, and QRS complexes at regular intervals. It also has a very regular rate of heartbeats, often between 60 and 100 per minute. This is known as the normal sinus rhythm (NSR). When a healthy heart is beating it is based on an impulse that originates in the atria and travels down the AV node and then propagates to the right and left bundle branches of His. The impulse then causes a rapid contraction of the ventricles. After a short delay, the ventricles repolarize and prepare for another impulse.

This process can be interrupted by abnormal depolarization sequences that can cause a broad QRS complex. This could be caused by a ventricular ectopic or a bundle branch block.

Symptoms of a broad QRS complex include shortness of breath and dizziness. Occasionally, the heart can become weak and stop beating altogether.

If you are a newbie, it can be helpful to use our free training module that provides a five-step ECG rhythm analysis method for quick learning to interpret EKG tracings. Once you have mastered the technique and become comfortable with it, you will be able to analyze most squiggly lines in an EKG paper.

Adult Heart Rate

In general, an irregular rhythm is more difficult to diagnose and will require more thorough evaluation and treatment. In addition, there may be more reversible causes of an irregular rhythm. Identifying and treating these reversible causes will allow the patient to get back on a more stable rhythm in the future.

Normal and Abnormal Heart Rate

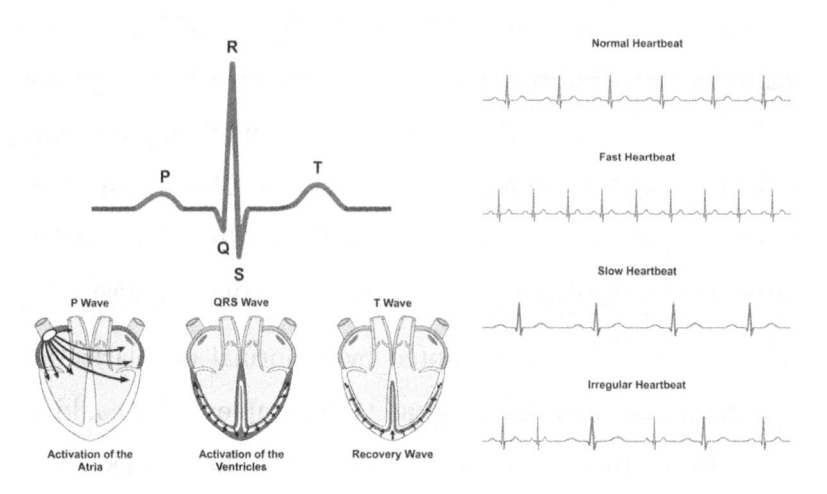

Bradycardia

Bradycardia is a slow heart rate, fewer than 60 beats per minute. It usually doesn't cause problems in most people, but a person with bradycardia may have symptoms like chest pain, dizziness, easy fatigue or shortness of breath.

The heart's normal rhythm is determined by the electrical signals that start each heartbeat and travel through the sinus node in the right atrium. When the signals from the sinus node are slowed or blocked, the heart's natural pacemaker becomes dysfunctional and the heart will beat too slowly. This type of bradycardia is known as sinus node-mediated bradycardia and can be transient or persistent.

Other factors can also cause bradycardia, such as low thyroid hormone levels and an electrolyte imbalance. Tests to check your blood for these conditions can help healthcare providers diagnose bradycardia.

Diagnosis: To diagnose bradycardia, health care providers use a combination of physical exams and tests to detect other conditions that can cause the heart to beat slowly. A healthcare provider might use a blood test to measure levels of thyroid hormones and a specialized protein called troponin. He or she may also perform a stress exercise test, which involves monitoring your heartbeat while you walk or ride a stationary bike.

A doctor can also take a detailed medical history and listen to your heart with a stethoscope. He or she will try to identify if the slow heartbeat is caused by any other medical conditions, such as a serious infection or an electrolyte imbalance.

Treatment: When the cause of your bradycardia isn't severe or if you're young, your healthcare provider might prescribe medications to control the symptoms and get your heart rate back to normal. These medications can include a beta-blocker, calcium-channel blocker or an anti-arrhythmia drug. They can also be used to treat the underlying condition that causes the bradycardia, such as low or high cholesterol or an electrolyte imbalance.

Pacemaker: When bradycardia is caused by a blocked sinus node or other abnormality in the heart, your doctor might recommend having a device (pacemaker) implanted under your skin. A pacemaker is a small, electrically connected device about the size of a matchbook that contains two leads. One lead is connected to the wall of your right atrium, while the other is attached to your right ventricle.

Your doctor might recommend a cardiologist to help determine the underlying cause of your bradycardia. The cardiologist can tell you what treatment is needed to fix your condition and how long you will need the medication.

The good news is that the prognosis for many people with bradycardia is improving. If the bradycardia is caused by underlying disorders, such as an electrolyte imbalance or low thyroid hormones, treatment can often relieve the symptoms and improve the person's quality of life.

What is Tachycardia?

Tachycardia, or tachyarrhythmia, is a fast heart rate (more than 100 beats per minute) that may be normal during exercise or when the body is stressed or it can be caused by an abnormal heart rhythm. Depending on the cause, tachycardia can cause problems with blood flow to the rest of the body and increase your risk of heart failure, sudden cardiac arrest or death.

Symptoms of Tachycardia

Some people with tachycardia have no symptoms and no complications develop, but others experience palpitations, dizziness or skipped heartbeats. These symptoms can be frightening or scary, but they are usually harmless if they are caught and treated early.

Identifying and Treating Tachycardia

Some types of tachycardia can be detected by your doctor using an electrocardiogram, or EKG. Often, a one-time office EKG will be enough to diagnose your condition. However, if your tachycardia isn't well controlled, you may need to wear a monitoring device called a Holter monitor for a period of time.

Sinus tachycardia is one of the most common types of tachycardia. It occurs when an electrical imbalance in the sinus node, the heart's natural pacemaker, causes the heart to beat too fast. Unlike paroxysmal supraventricular tachycardia (PSVT), which has no warning signs, sinus tachycardia can be dangerous, especially when it happens in conjunction with other symptoms. It can be a sign of serious disease, such as sepsis or shock. It can also be a symptom of a heart disorder or other problem, such as thyroid disease.

It can be difficult to diagnose because the P wave morphology and the setting in which it occurs vary from patient to patient. Diagnosis is based on the ECG and whether or not there is an atrial ventricular relationship of 1 or >1. In addition, narrow-QRS complex tachycardia suggests that anterograde conduction occurs through the atrioventricular node and His-Purkinje system, while wide-QRS complex tachycardia indicates ventricular activation.

The atrial ventricular relationship of 1 is the most helpful, but not necessarily exclusive, in differentiating sinus tachycardia from ventricular tachycardia. This is not a reliable predictor of the underlying etiology, however.

A patient's age, race and gender should be considered as a clinical predictor of tachycardia. Patients who have a family history of tachycardia are at higher risk for developing it.

Some tachycardias can be treated with medication or surgery, such as radio ablation, which involves injecting radioactive material into tiny areas of the heart that cause electrical signal problems. Other treatments involve lifestyle changes or more advanced methods of treating tachycardia.

Your doctor will recommend a course of treatment, which will depend on the type and severity of your tachycardia. In some cases, your tachycardia can be permanently corrected with a device called an implantable cardioverter defibrillator or a leadless pacemaker.

What is Atrial Fibrillation?

Atrial fibrillation (AFib) is an irregular, quivery heartbeat that can cause clots, stroke and other complications. It is one of the most common heart rhythm problems and affects 2.7 million Americans. When these cells fire abnormally, your heartbeat changes to an irregular, fluttery beat that doesn't move blood to the lower chambers (ventricles).

Normally, the electrical impulses in the atria send signals to your lower chambers to start a normal heartbeat. In a normal, healthy heart, the electrical signal that starts a heartbeat comes from your sinus node in the upper right chamber of your heart. Your sinus node is also known as your natural pacemaker.

When the sinus node signals the atria to start a normal heartbeat, your muscles contract and squeeze to move blood out of the atria and into the ventricles. Your heart also relaxes between contractions, so the atria can be filled with blood again and your body can get enough oxygen.

Your body needs the right amount of oxygen to work properly, so it pumps a steady flow of blood to the rest of your body. If your body doesn't have enough oxygen, you may feel tired or lightheaded.

Risk factors for AF include age, heart disease and high blood pressure. Other conditions that can increase the risk of developing AF include diabetes, a thyroid disorder, lung disease and some medicines.

The goal of treatment is to reduce your risk of clots, which can lead to heart failure and stroke. It's usually placed under your skin and will send small bursts of electricity to your heart when it beats too slowly.

A holder monitor or portable event monitor can be used to check your heartbeat. This device records your heartbeat for several days and gives your doctor a chance to spot irregularities.

There is also a blood test that can show if you have potassium or thyroid problems and how well your liver and kidneys are working. These tests can be very important in helping your provider treat you with the right medicine.

Chapter 4.
ECG Ischemia and Infarction

When the blood supply to the heart muscle is diminished, a condition called myocardial ischemia develops. This may be transmural (affecting the entire thickness of the myocardium) or subendocardial, affecting only the innermost part of the myocardium, the heart's inner endocardium.

Myocardial infarction is generally the result of severe ischemia, but it can also occur when a coronary artery is blocked but the blockage is not complete. Infarctions can be localized, affecting a single lead, or widespread, involving the entire left ventricle. Inferior wall infarctions are sometimes referred to as "anteroseptal" or "strictly anterior," whereas anterior wall infarctions are often referred to as "antero-lateral or apical."

The diagnosis of MI is usually based on the characteristic changes seen in multiple contiguous leads, as well as the presence of Q waves. In addition, many patients with AMI have symptoms of the disease, which can help to differentiate it from ischemia.

This infarction may be caused by a coronary artery obstruction, but is more likely to result from a ventricular aneurysm or other pathology that affects the ventricular septum. The most common clinical signs of myocardial infarction are pain, shortness of breath, and hypertension. However, many patients with AMI have little or no symptoms and therefore are not able to report them. Consequently, the characteristic ECG changes seen in patients with AMI can be missed or mistaken for ischemia.

ECG Ischemia and Infarction

The ECG has a very important role in the diagnosis and management of ischemia and infarction. It is an invaluable tool for the early detection of acute coronary syndromes, and it is used to assess the prognosis of patients with chest pain. It also aids in the identification of patients at high risk of developing a cardiac event.

a. Overview of ECG ischemia and infarction

The most common form of ischemia is transmural, which occurs when the blood flow to the heart muscle is reduced due to a blockage in a coronary artery. It is usually associated with unstable angina.

It can also be caused by subendocardial ischemia, which occurs when the blood flow to the ventricular wall is reduced because of a blockage in a coronary branch. This form of ischemia causes the T waves to become inverted or flattened, and can produce a biphasic T wave pattern. It is often seen in leads V1 to V3, and it can lead to an accelerated onset of chest pain.

b. Overview of ECG infarction

Myocardial infarction is the most frequent cause of chest pain, occurring in 50 to 90% of cases. It is the most serious type of cardiovascular disease, and it can be fatal. However, it can also be treatable with medicines or a procedure called angioplasty.

c. Overview of ECG ischemic symptoms

Chest pain is usually worse when you exercise, but it can be felt at rest or while you are sleeping.

d. Overview of ECG infarct changes

Ischemia and infarction produce a wide range of changes on the ECG, with most affecting the ST segment. Changes can be subtle or dramatic, and are usually recorded in the first 12 hours after the onset of chest pain. Various diagnostic scoring systems have been developed to improve the sensitivity of the ECG in detecting myocardial infarction. 58 These are not foolproof, and may not be able to exclude left ventricular hypertrophy or other conditions that cause ST/T wave changes but do not result in chest pain. Several new technologies are now available that can monitor cardiac activity in real time, providing rapid diagnosis of chest pain and reducing the delay in treatment of ischemia.

e. Overview of ECG infarct patterns

The first ECG infarct pattern, known as the wellens syndrome, is caused by a proximal LAD artery occlusion. It usually has a broad pattern of widespread ST depression (leads I, II and aVF) with small Q waves in some of the leads, and a biphasic T wave pattern in the anterior chest leads. The T wave area curve (TWAC) is a characteristic morphology of this pattern, and it has a strong correlation with ischemic heart disease.

f. Overview of ECG infarction in children

Acute myocardial infarction can cause a range of symptoms in young people, including chest pain and a racing heart. The chest pain is most often in the center of the chest and may be severe or mild.

Ischemia and Infarction

Ischemia: a decrease in the blood flow to a particular organ or part of an organ (heart muscle) due to blockage of the blood vessels supplying that area.

Atherosclerosis: Atherosclerosis is the thickening of the arteries that carries blood to the heart, due to deposition of fatty material such as cholesterol. This artery narrowing causes atherosclerosis, a condition that increases the risk of cardiovascular events such as stroke and heart attack. Coronary artery disease: The main form of ischemic heart disease is coronary artery disease, or CHD. The arteries that carry blood to the heart muscle are narrowed by the buildup of plaque, which contains fatty materials such as cholesterol and clots that can obstruct the blood flow. The clots can rupture, causing an infarction or heart attack.

Angiography: It is useful for assessing the size and shape of blood vessels. It can also reveal abnormalities such as narrowing, thrombosis, or spasm.

CT Findings That Are Early Indicators of Ischemia and Infarction:

Atherosclerotic plaque occlusion in the left anterior descending artery is the most common site of ischemia, although a large occlusion of the right coronary artery is also common. During exercise, the plaque narrows the coronary artery by as much as 75% and the reduced oxygen supply can cause angina pectoris or stable ischemic chest pain that resolves when cardiac contractility returns to normal.

Clinical presentation is dependent on the etiology of the ischemia and may include pain, pallor, and hypothermia. The earliest neurologic signs of vascular insufficiency are subjective sensory deficits such as numbness, paresthesia, and paralysis in the lower extremities. These symptoms are the six Ps of ischemia and are often first exhibited in the lower extremity, particularly in the anterior compartment of the limb.

Pulses: Acute limb ischemia usually shows severely decreased pulses. However, if pulses are normal in the asymptomatic contralateral extremity, then this reflects chronic arterial occlusion that has not triggered the acute ischemia.

Electrocardiographic changes: Ischemia often produces ST depressions in multiple leads on the ECG, whereas myocardial infarction usually produces ST elevations in only one lead. Ischemia also typically does not result in Q waves, whereas myocardial infarction typically does.

In ischemic strokes, a decrease in oxygen supply prevents the formation of ATP, which is the metabolic energy required for cellular function. This decrease in ATP production also leads to a reduction in phosphorylation of DNA, which is essential for cytokines and other biochemical signaling. In addition, a decrease in oxidative phosphorylation of proteins reduces the production of amino acids and other key molecules that are important for cell growth and differentiation. Hence, the ischemia that occurs during a stroke can lead to apoptosis, or cell death.

ECG Differential Diagnosis of Ischemia and Infarction

The electrocardiogram (ECG) is an invaluable clinical diagnostic tool that can be used to differentiate between different cardiac disorders, including chest pain.

Diagnosis

The position of exploring electrodes may influence the sensitivity of the ECG for ischemia detection. Small infarcts or areas of ischemic ischemia that are electrically "silent" are unlikely to produce abnormal Q waves, and are therefore likely to be missed.

However, the pathological substrate of these Q waves is uncertain, and they are not useful in diagnosing an established myocardial infarction (MI) if they are accompanied by other ECG changes that are unrelated to myocardial ischemia, such as a T-wave inversion or ST-segment elevation in one or more leads. The most common ECG changes in myocardial ischemia are T-wave tenting or inversion, ST-segment depression, and J-point elevation in one or more leads.

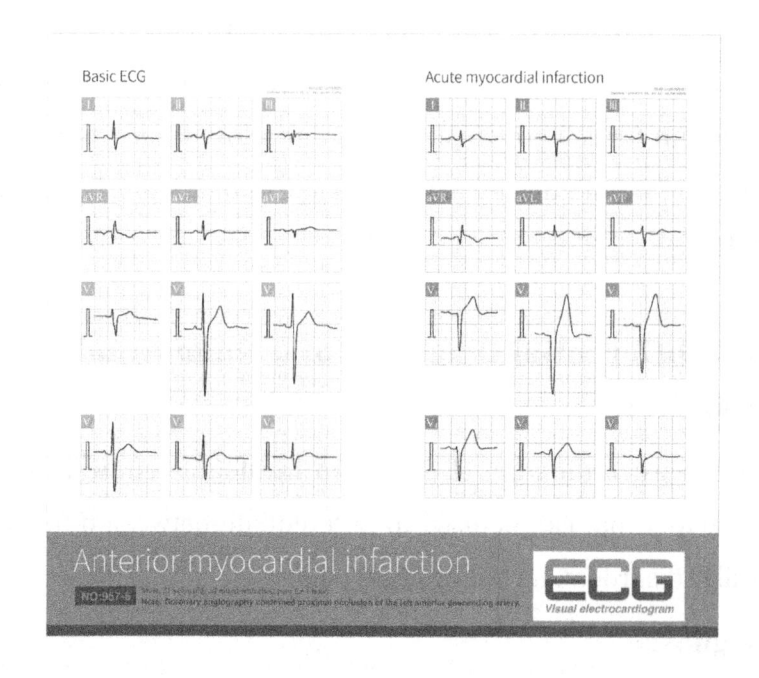

ECG diagnosis of infarction

The conventional ECG approach to the diagnosis of myocardial infarction is limited by the sensitivity of the ECG for detecting AMI. Currently, the sensitivity of the ECG to detect AMI is around 50% in patients with chest pain.

Several studies have demonstrated that a 12-lead ECG with NSR (negative ST segment elevation in three or more leads) is significantly more likely to diagnose NSTEMI than an ECG without NSR.

This sensitivity is not fixed, and it is expected to improve with the development of higher-resolution technologies for real-time cardiac monitoring. This could vastly improve the sensitivity of the ECG for identifying myocardial ischemia and infarction and thus allow more targeted therapies to be delivered quickly.

Diagnosis of infarction involves a thorough evaluation of the patient's clinical history and examination, in combination with an ECG and serial cardiac enzymes and other laboratory tests. This holistic approach is essential in avoiding the misinterpretation of findings, and in guiding treatment.

The development of higher-resolution technologies for the ECG has been very promising, with a growing emphasis on dynamic as opposed to fixed changes. This is believed to greatly improve the sensitivity of the ECG to detect ischemia and infarction, particularly in cases of non-ST-elevation myocardial infarction, but there is a need to refine these new techniques to ensure that they are used with care. This would benefit patients, as it is likely to reduce the amount of time they spend in hospital and improve their quality of life and outcome.

Management of ECG Ischemia and Infarction

Although a variety of tests can be used to diagnose these disorders, the ECG remains the most reliable and sensitive test. Acute myocardial infarction (MI) is defined as ischemic destruction of myocardium that is caused by the obstruction of one or more coronary arteries. This occurs in approximately 1.0

million Americans per year and results in death for 300,000 to 400,000 individuals. In most cases, the damage is localized to a single segment of myocardium, but it can also be transmural, which involves the entire thickness of the heart muscle.

During an infarction, blood flow to the damaged area is cut off and the tissue becomes dead (necrotic). This necrosis can be seen on an ECG, where there are abnormal ST segments or T waves. In the most severe cases of infarction, the heart's ability to pump blood is reduced or blocked entirely and cardiogenic shock develops, leading to death.

Myocardial infarction can occur as a transmural (into the entire thickness of the heart) or subendocardial (into the inner part of the heart, below the endocardium) infarct. During transmural infarcts, the myocardium is destroyed completely, whereas in subendocardial infarcts, the heart muscle is partially damaged.

Cardiac electrocardiography is an important diagnostic tool for the detection of ischemia and infarction, but it has limitations. For example, ST depressions can be caused by a non-cardiac cause and are not as sensitive for detecting infarction as are Q wave changes, especially if the Q waves are persistent.

QRS amplitudes are also often a poor indicator of infarction because they can be misleading for assessing risk. In addition, a patient with an infarct can have no change in the QRS amplitudes for long periods, and a small infarct can have an enormous amplitude.

The sensitivity of the ECG for detecting infarcts has been improved by using complex scoring systems that require ST or T wave criteria, as well as QRS scoring thresholds. These algorithms have been applied to clinical practice and have greatly increased sensitivity for diagnosing an acute myocardial infarction compared to traditional methods of ECG evaluation.

However, despite these improvements, most infarcts are still fatal. The mortality rate for patients who survive initial hospitalization is 8 to 10%, with most deaths occurring within the first 6 weeks of infarction.

Emergency intervention during an episode of chest pain is the primary way to reduce morbidity and mortality in patients with suspected MI. This includes intravenous fluids, oxygen administration, and continuous single-lead ECG monitoring.

An early diagnosis of an infarct on the ECG is essential to assess patient outcome and guide revascularization. This decision can be made by measuring cardiac markers, such as CK elevation and cardiac troponins.

Revascularization can be attempted through thrombolysis, angioplasty, and/or invasive coronary intervention.

Chapter 5.
ECG Arrhythmias

Arrhythmias are abnormalities of the heart's rhythm that cause an increased risk for cardiac complications, which in turn increase the patient's chances of dying. These arrhythmias include atrial fibrillation (AF), sinus tachycardia, supraventricular tachycardia and ventricular tachycardia.

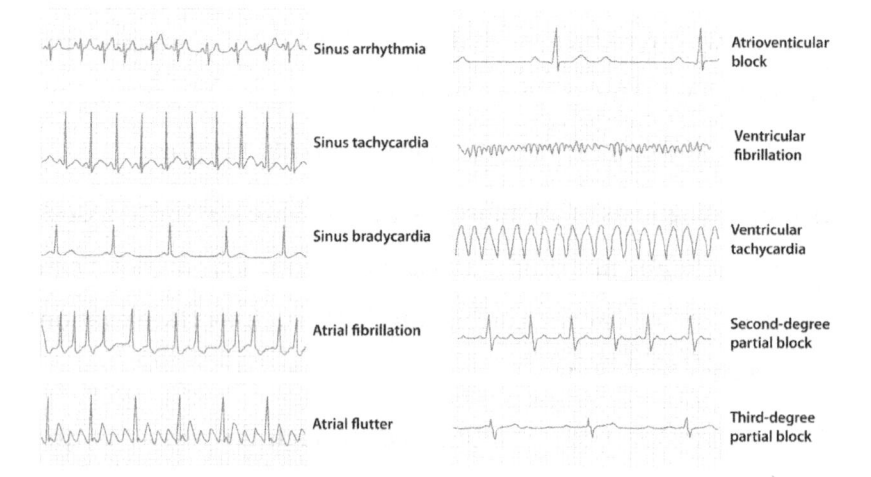

~~	Sinus arrhythmia	~~~	Atrioventicular block
~~	Sinus tachycardia	~~~	Ventricular fibrillation
~~	Sinus bradycardia	~~~	Ventricular tachycardia
~~	Atrial fibrillation	~~~	Second-degree partial block
~~	Atrial flutter	~~~	Third-degree partial block

There are many possible causes for arrhythmias. These can be primary (i.e., caused by changes in the heart's electrical system) or secondary (i.e., resulting from outside factors that alter the heart's electrical system).

The most common arrhythmia is AF. It is caused by disorganized electrical activity of the atria and AV node. The atria depolarize rapidly and the AV node responds by slowing conduction down to the ventricles. This protective mechanism works very well unless the AV node is damaged or the person is taking certain medications that inhibit AV nodal conduction, such as beta blockers, digitalis or calcium channel blockers.

A typical AF ECG shows multiple reentrant flutter waves in lead II and aVF.

Management: If the patient is not asymptomatic and the arrhythmia is not life-threatening, it should be managed with antiarrhythmic medication such as beta-blockers or digitalis. Other therapies may be required if the underlying cause is serious or cannot be controlled with antiarrhythmic medications.

Electrophysiologic Study: This is the most important step in interpreting the ECG rhythm strip. This is where you correlate the information that you have gathered in steps 1 through 6 with your knowledge of the heart's electrophysiology. This will help you make the best initial decisions in treating your patient's symptoms and potential heart problems.

Whether you are a nurse or an intensivist, you should be able to interpret the rhythm strip in the same manner that a physician would. However, it is essential to be able to remember the six basic steps for interpreting the rhythm strip because this will give you the necessary skills to quickly assess your patient's health and begin medical interventions.

Overview of ECG Arrhythmias

Arrhythmias occur when the electrical signals that send messages from the brain to the heart don't work correctly. These abnormal heart rhythms are usually harmless but can cause serious complications if they are not treated.

In a normal heart, the electrical signals travel from the brain to the heart through the sinus node and then through the heart's upper chambers (atria). When they arrive at the ventricles, they slow down so that they can fill with blood and pump it to the lungs or to the rest of the body.

A normal resting heart rate is 60 to 100 beats per minute. But the heart's rate can be too fast, too slow or erratic.

The quickest way to determine if you have an arrhythmia is with a simple, painless test called electrocardiography (ECG). Your doctor will place a small lead in your chest and use a machine to record your heart's electrical activity.

An ECG can pick up a wide range of problems, including arrhythmias. Some arrhythmias are so brief that they don't change the resting heart rate much, but others can last for hours.

If the standard ECG doesn't detect an arrhythmia, your doctor may order another test that can catch them quickly. One type is a Holter monitor, which records the heart for a day or longer to see if an arrhythmia occurs. An alternative is an event monitor, which you wear for a week or longer and switch on when you experience symptoms.

Aside from an ECG, a heart specialist can also do an echocardiogram and a tilt table test. These tests can help determine if an arrhythmia is triggered by exercise or exertion and whether a medication is needed.

Medications for mild and infrequent arrhythmias often involve less frequent doses of medications or changes in dosages. They might include a blood pressure-lowering drug, a diuretic, a calcium channel blocker and a beta-blocker.

Other drugs might be used to treat more severe and frequent arrhythmias.

Suppose a medication is not effective in controlling the arrhythmia. In that case, your healthcare provider may recommend surgical ablation, which uses a thin tube to destroy or remove parts of the heart that are causing the problem. This is done in a hospital setting and is usually only used when other treatments have failed.

Your GP can also refer you to a specialist, who will prescribe a variety of medications and devices for treating your arrhythmia. They might also want to do a stress test or tilt table test.

Types of ECG Arrhythmias

Arrhythmias are disturbances in the normal rhythm of your heart. They are caused by problems with the way your heart sends out electrical signals that coordinate the contraction of your upper and lower heart chambers to pump blood around your body.

In a healthy heart, the heart's electrical system works normally. These signals go through a series of pathways that lead from your sinus node (situated in the upper part of your chest) to your ventricles (the lower chambers of your heart). They then move through a cluster of cells called the AV node, which slows them down so they can fill your ventricles with blood.

When these electrical impulses arrive in your ventricles, they trigger the contraction of your heart muscle to pump blood into your lungs or the rest of your body. These signals also tell your heart when it's time to stop and start again.

Once your heart is filled with blood, it pumps the blood to the lungs to be oxygenated and to the rest of your body through your veins.

Problems with this signaling process can result in abnormal heart rhythms that are asymptomatic or cause symptoms, such a weakening or fluttering feeling in your chest, shortness of breath or weakness. They can also be a sign of a serious health problem.

These heartbeats can be grouped into two categories: bradyarrhythmias and tachyarrhythmias, based on where the abnormal heartbeats start in the heart and how they affect your resting heart rate. Doctors also group them by how they affect your heart's ability to pump blood, including whether they start in the ventricles or the atria.

Atrial tachycardia is an early extra beat in the atrium (the upper chambers of your heart). It's usually harmless, but it may cause long-term complications if you have other conditions.

This type of heartbeat can be triggered by stress, strenuous exercise or certain stimulants, such as caffeine and nicotine. It can also be a warning sign of a serious heart condition, such as atrial fibrillation, which is an irregular beating in the upper chambers of your heart.

Ventricular tachycardia is an extra fast heartbeat that originates in the ventricles of your heart. It can be dangerous if it lasts for more than 30 minutes or if it is accompanied by chest pain.

These types of heartbeats are a sign that you have an abnormal heart rhythm and need medical treatment to fix it. Your doctor will check your blood pressure, heart rate, and other heart-related symptoms before deciding on the best course of treatment for you. They may recommend medications, lifestyle changes, invasive therapies or surgery.

Electrocardiogram Findings in Arrhythmias

Electrocardiogram (ECG) findings in arrhythmias are a common concern for doctors and other health care professionals. These findings can reveal underlying heart disease or abnormal heart rhythms that need to be monitored and treated. Fortunately, many of these conditions can be identified using an ECG.

A 12-lead ECG can be used to look for abnormalities in the heart's electrical signals, which cause it to beat too fast or too slow. It can also be used to map the spread of these signals, so a doctor can identify and treat an arrhythmia before it causes serious problems.

The test involves placing up to 12 sensors (electrodes) on your chest and arms and a monitor to record the signals that make your heart beat. The electrodes can be sticky patches that are attached to your skin, or they can be a small tube that is tipped with electrodes and threaded through your blood vessels.

An ECG is important for diagnosing a variety of health issues, including heart attacks and other heart problems, strokes and infections. It can also be used to assess whether or not you have certain conditions, such as diabetes or high cholesterol, that increase your risk for developing an arrhythmia.

Sinus tachycardia: This is an abnormal heart rate that occurs only in the sinus node (the part of the heart that produces electrical impulses and sends them to the ventricles). This condition is more common in infants, young people, anxious people and those who are extremely tired or depressed.

This can happen for a variety of reasons, such as high or low blood pressure, stress or certain medications. The SA node may be damaged, or the conduction pathway that carries the impulses from your brain to your heart may be interrupted or blocked.

The ECG can be normal if your sinus node works normally, and all of the heart's beats are normal. However, this rhythm may be a problem in some conditions, such as if you're an athlete or on certain medications or if it gets so slow that it causes symptoms like fainting or dizziness.

Bradycardia: This is a very slow heart rate that occurs when the natural pacemaker in your heart's sinoatrial node (SA node) is not working correctly, or the impulse that sends it to your heart's ventricles is interrupted or blocked. It is often caused by high blood pressure, diabetes or stress.

These arrhythmias are called bradyarrhythmias because they occur when your heart's rate is slow, or when your heart's natural pacemaker, the sinus node, is not working correctly. The most common bradyarrhythmias are AV block, atrial fibrillation and atrial flutter.

Treatment options for these heart rhythms vary based on your individual situation, but they can include medication and catheter ablation of the area that's causing the problem. Implantable cardioverter-defibrillators are another option for treating arrhythmias that are a danger to your life.

Management of ECG Arrhythmias

The ability to manage ECG arrhythmias is a skill that is essential for nurses working in critical care settings. Nurses are the first clinicians who should look at the ECG and be able to identify abnormalities in order to activate appropriate emergency health teams and initiate early interventions that may prevent serious complications and death.

A variety of studies have shown that a number of nurses do not have adequate knowledge in relation to the initial management of cardiac arrhythmias and are often unable to recognize and manage an episode of ventricular tachycardia, which can result in life-threatening conditions if left untreated. This study aimed to determine the level of competency in ECG interpretation among nurses and how it is related to their ability to identify ventricular tachycardia and to manage it.

Chapter 6.
ECG Myocardial Ischemia

Myocardial ischemia can cause a variety of changes to the ECG.

These include ST segment elevation and depression, alternans (ST-T waves that change in amplitude from upright to negative or inverted) and intraventricular conduction abnormalities such as the U-wave inversion.

ST Segment Elevation and Depression

This elevation of the ST segment occurs because ischemia alters the electrical properties of the heart tissue, leading to voltage gradients between normal myocardial tissue and ischemic myocardial tissue that create injury currents in the heart cells. These injury currents can elevate or depress the ST segment and are thus a significant diagnostic feature of ischemic heart disease.

Interventricular Conduction Abnormalities

The conduction system is a critical component of cardiac physiology and is responsible for the generation of the action potential. Ischemia alters the conduction system by causing changes in the repolarization of the ventricular myocytes and their membrane potentials, and may also lead to changes in the timing of the conduction cycle. The resulting ECG changes are called intraventricular conduction abnormalities and occur primarily in the inferior leads on an ECG.

Intraventricular conduction abnormalities, especially those associated with STEMI, are very common in patients with myocardial ischemia and can be very difficult to diagnose. However, they can be helpful in predicting an impending MI or chest pain.

Alternans

The alternans on an ECG are characteristic of ischemic heart disease and are present in most cases of obstructive coronary artery disease. They are present in two or more ECG leads and are usually dynamic (appearing and disappearing during periods of asymptomatic cardiovascular activity).

Hyperacute T-waves

These symmetric, broad based and high amplitude T-waves are seen immediately after occlusion of the coronary artery and occur when ischemia reaches the epicardial heart tissue. They are characterized by their rapid onset, relatively short duration and disappearance within seconds.

Hyperacute T-waves are also seen in patients with transmural ischemia, a type of ischemic cardiomyopathy, and can be found in a greater number of ECG leads than ischemic ST-segment elevations.

They are characterized by increased potassium concentrations, which increase the repolarization of the ventricular cells and cause them to become more sensitive to changes in ion voltage. They are seen in most cases of obstructive CAD and are a critical diagnostic feature of ischemic CAD.

Q Waves

In addition to ST-segment elevation and depression, the ischemic ECG may also display broad negative deflections known as Q waves. These are produced by injury currents originating from the ischemic heart tissue and can appear in the anterior wall of the left ventricle on an ECG.

Although these are commonly viewed as an ECG sign of myocardial ischemia, they can be a hallmark of any serious underlying cardiovascular problem. For example, they can occur in the context of pericarditis and in severe chronic obstructive pulmonary disease, which can be life-threatening.

What Are the Signs and Symptoms of Ischemia?

Ischemia (i-SHEH-meh-muh-she-mEEK) is a term that describes a reduction in blood flow to one part of the body. It can affect any tissue or organ, and can cause a shortage of oxygen for normal cellular function.

Signs and symptoms vary depending on the type of ischemia, but usually a patient will have chest pain when it occurs. This pain can occur with or without activity and sometimes it's accompanied by other signs of cardiac problems such as shortness of breath, nausea or vomiting.

The pain may start suddenly, or it can come and go over time. Symptoms also can include chest tightness, dizziness, weakness and trouble breathing.

Symptoms can get worse with age, but they can also be relieved by taking medications and following your doctor's instructions. In severe cases, you might need surgery to improve blood flow to the heart or reduce your risk of a heart attack.

Intestinal Ischemia/Mesenteric Ischemia

Ischemic bowel disease is a condition that can be caused by a blockage in the blood vessels supplying the intestines. This blockage can happen in the stomach, small intestines or large intestines. In addition, it can be triggered by conditions such as atherosclerosis, arrhythmias, hernias or kidney or spleen disease.

Athletes with ischemic bowel disease can have difficulty exercising and may experience fatigue and numbness. In severe cases, they can't perform their favorite sports and may even lose weight.

Silent ischemia is another common problem, especially among people who have had a heart attack or diabetes. This plaque collects in the arteries, narrowing them and blocking the passage of blood to the heart or brain.

Occasionally, this buildup can rupture and form a blood clot in the artery. This can happen when a person is at high risk for ischemic stroke, such as if they have a family history of this condition or are older than 65.

Other causes of ischemia include high cholesterol, obesity, diabetes and a certain kind of abnormal heart rhythm known as atrial fibrillation. This disorder causes the heart to beat too fast, leading to a reduction in oxygen supply and causing irregularities in the heart's rhythm.

How Do You Fix Myocardial Ischemia?

Causes of myocardial ischemia include a buildup of plaque inside your coronary arteries that narrows the artery and blocks blood flow. The plaque is made of cholesterol and other substances that clog the arteries over time. A buildup of this plaque, also called atherosclerosis, is the main cause of ischemic heart disease and is responsible for about 70% of fatal heart attacks.

Ischemia causes symptoms such as chest pain and discomfort that get worse with activity. If a blockage is small, it can be treated with medicine. But if it's large and close to the heart, your doctor may recommend a procedure called angioplasty or stent placement. The procedure involves inserting a catheter or stent through an artery to reopen the artery and improve blood flow to your heart.

Your doctor will tell you what treatment works best for you.

The goal of myocardial ischemia treatment is to reduce your risk of a heart attack or stroke and prevent the condition from returning in the future. To do this, you'll need to eliminate or change the risk factors that put you at greater risk for a heart attack.

You should also get a regular checkup from your doctor, especially if you're a smoker or if you have high blood pressure or high cholesterol. Your doctor will give you a physical exam, perform tests and run blood tests to look for signs of heart damage.

Getting adequate amounts of sleep, reducing stress and taking care of yourself during recovery are all part of your treatment plan. A healthy lifestyle is one of the most effective ways to treat myocardial ischemia and prevent it from developing in the future.

The difference between heart attack and ischemia

Ischemia is a lack of oxygenated blood flow to the heart muscle. It usually occurs when one or more coronary arteries are blocked by the build-up of plaque. When plaque builds up, it blocks or restricts the flow of blood to your heart, leading to a heart attack.

Signs: Feeling weak or dizzy; breaking out into a cold sweat.

You might also have a sudden, severe pain in your stomach that spreads to your chest or back. The pain may be worse when you stand or sit up.

A clot that breaks free from the plaque in a coronary artery and floats to your heart may block blood flow to your heart, causing a heart attack. A clot can also form in the arteries that bring blood to your brain (brain arteries), causing a stroke.

What is the treatment for myocardial ischemia?

Ischemia is most often treated by improving your heart's blood flow and making healthy lifestyle choices. This includes maintaining a healthy weight, reducing your stress level and eating a diet low in saturated fats, trans fats and sugar. It also means avoiding smoking and limiting alcohol use.

Some people are at risk for silent ischemia, which is a lack of oxygen-rich blood flow to the heart without any chest pain or other symptoms. Silent ischemia can be caused by many things, such as heart disease and atherosclerosis, but the most common is the build-up of plaque in your arteries. Other risk factors for heart disease can also lead to ischemic episodes, including high cholesterol levels and obesity.

What is the difference between a heart attack and a heart arrest?

A heart attack is the most serious type of ischemic episode. It is also the most likely to cause death or lead to hospitalization, although it does not always occur immediately.

What is the difference between ischemic heart disease and myocardial infarction?

Ischemic heart disease refers to the condition where blood flow is reduced to the heart, preventing it from receiving enough oxygen. It can be caused by coronary artery disease, a narrowing of the arteries that supply blood to your heart, and sometimes by a blood clot or spasm in the arteries.

What Are ECG Tools?

An ECG Tool is a device that records the electrical activity of the heart. This information can help doctors diagnose and monitor various cardiac conditions, such as a heart attack, tachycardia (rapid heart rate), arrhythmia (irregular heartbeat) and heart failure.

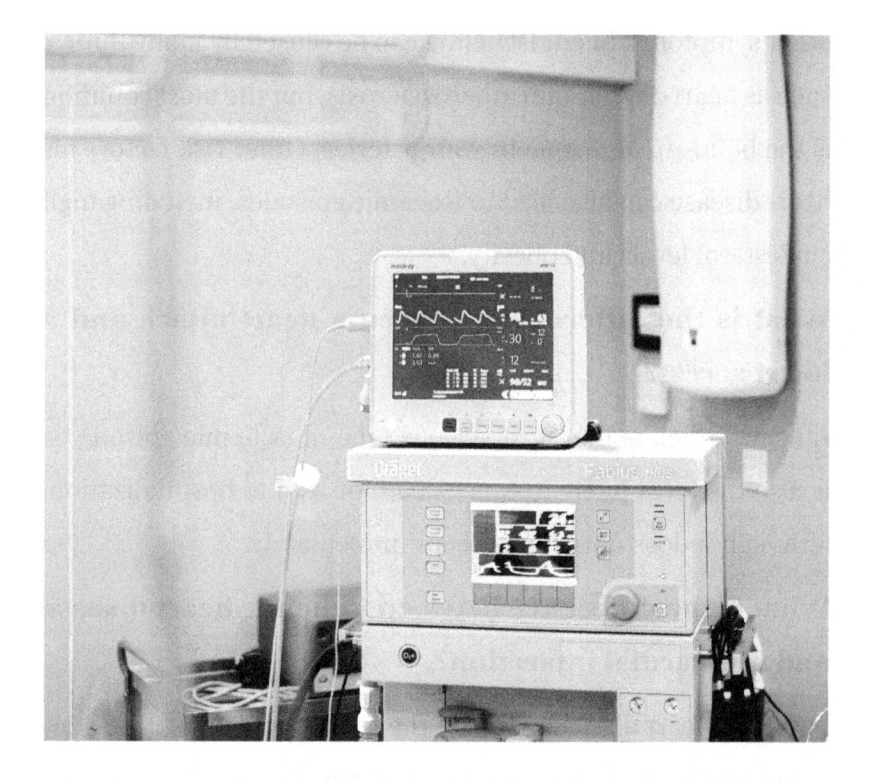

ECG Tools are used in hospitals, clinics and private practices to record a patient's heart activity. These devices range from basic ECG machines to sophisticated medical-grade instruments that are equipped with advanced software and specialized features to provide healthcare professionals with a complete view of any patient's condition.

A standard electrocardiogram is a quick and easy test that can identify several types of abnormalities. This test is performed in a hospital or doctor's office and is commonly done to help detect cardiac conditions, including arrhythmia and irregular heartbeats.

During an ECG, a medical professional uses up to 12 electrodes that are attached to specific areas of the body. These sticky patches are connected to a computer that records and interprets the signals that make up the electrical activity of the heart.

After the ECG, your care provider will show you the tracing on a special monitor or paper and explain what it means. They'll also take your temperature and check your blood pressure.

A doctor can also recommend an ECG monitor that you can wear 24 hours a day for a period of time, called a Holter monitor. This monitor records the tracing for up to two days, and your doctor can compare the results with other tests that you get later on.

The Holter monitor is most often recommended if you have symptoms that indicate that something might be wrong with your heart. This includes sudden, irregular heartbeats or palpitations, shortness of breath and dizziness.

Your doctor can use the results of a holder monitor to monitor your heart for up to two weeks, and they can also check if you are having a heart attack or other life-threatening problem. These devices can also be used to track your heart rhythm before and after you have certain procedures, such as surgery or a cardiac catheterization.

Many people have personal-use ECG monitors at home to track their heart rhythm and rate. These devices are not as accurate as the ECGs that your doctor uses in the hospital or their office, but they can still be useful for checking your heart's rhythm and rate. Some of these monitors are more sensitive than others, so they might pick up very small changes in your heart's rhythm.

Chapter 7.
Emergency Situations

Despite the importance of the ECG, many medical professionals do not have a complete understanding of how it works or the rules that must be followed to interpret an ECG. This can lead to errors in ECG interpretation and poor outcomes for patients.

Cardiac Monitoring System

The cardiac monitoring system used in emergency departments includes an ECG generator, ECG monitor and specialized paper that records an ECG at a speed of 25 mm/second. The specialized paper is a thin, translucent sheet that allows the physician to see the ECG as it is being recorded on it.

A standard ECG is made up of five electrodes connected by a series of wires to form a lead configuration. This is called the "standard three lead" or "Einthoven's triangle". The red electrode is placed on the left lateral base of the chest, while the green and blue wires connect to the other two electrodes.

ECG Components

Each ECG component is usually labelled and will have its own name. This is to make it easier for the clinician to understand the ECG and identify which component may be the cause of the abnormality in the patient's condition.

Waves

A wave is a change in electrical potential that occurs in cardiac cells when a voltage change takes place to the cell membranes. There are a number of different types of waves but the most common wave is the P wave that represents the depolarization of the atrial cells and the QRS complex that represents ventricular depolarization.

QRS Complex

The QRS complex is a very important ECG component as it is the originating point of an electrical impulse and the location from which that impulse travels to other parts of the heart. This is why the width of the QRS complex is often a significant criterion for rapid ECG interpretation.

The direction of the waveforms is another important factor. Typically, the shortest and tallest amplitude of an ECG wave will be a result of depolarization that is travelling towards the positive electrode. This can result in an upright waveform that resembles the P wave or it can be the opposite with a depolarizing wave that is travelling away from the positive electrode.

Overview of ECG in Emergency Situations

An ECG is a way of detecting heart problems by recording the electrical activity of your heart. This can help doctors diagnose and treat heart conditions. It's used to diagnose abnormalities such as enlargement of the heart, abnormal heart rhythms or damage to the heart's main electrical system (cardiac arrhythmia).

Getting an ECG is not painful.

A nurse, doctor or ECG technician will take an ECG of your heart using electrodes that are attached to your chest, arms and legs. The electrodes connect to a machine that takes the reading and sends it to your doctor. You'll be asked to lie still for a few minutes, and you can't do anything special to prepare for the test.

Your body has many different kinds of electrical signals that are sent from your heart to your brain, skin and other parts of the body. These electrical signals don't travel evenly over your skin, so the device compares them and measures the strength of the signal from each of 12 leads - that's why it's called a 12-lead ECG.

The ECG can pick up on small electrical changes in your heart muscles that cause pulsating waves of electricity to travel from your heart to the electrodes on your skin. These waves of electricity are very tiny, so it's important to use a very high-quality ECG equipment.

Electrocardiograms are sensitive and accurate.

An ECG can help to identify cardiac rhythm abnormalities, conduction problems and channelopathies, such as long QT syndrome and Brugada syndrome, which may indicate heart disease. It can also help to detect a heart attack and assess the extent of damage.

a. Overview of ECG in emergency situations

The American College of Cardiology and the American Heart Association recommend that all patients presenting to the emergency department with chest pain/anginal equivalent symptoms receive an initial ECG within 10 minutes of presentation. However, in a large contemporary sample of ambulance-presented patients, only 59% received an initial ECG within this time.

Consequently, in order to comply with the American Heart Association's recommendation for a prompt ECG, a number of strategies are required to improve ECG screening in the ambulance setting. Firstly, all ambulance crews should be trained to obtain an ECG of their patient within 10 minutes of a call for a suspected ischemic episode. Secondly, emergency nurses should be trained to recognize and triage patients with ischemic symptoms as soon as possible.

ECG in Cardiac Arrest

An electrocardiogram (ECG or EKG) is a test that checks the electrical activity of your heart. It is quick, painless and non-invasive. It can show changes in the electrical activity of the heart that increase your risk of sudden death from cardiac arrest, or abnormalities that can affect a person's health.

Your doctor will usually recommend an ECG if you are at risk of heart disease, or if you have certain conditions. You may also need an ECG to check the effects of certain medications on your heart.

The ECG detects tiny electrical changes on the skin that occur during heart muscle depolarization or repolarization. These waves are recorded by a special machine called an electrocardiograph (ECG).

You need to remove all clothing that can interfere with the electrodes, including shirts and blouses. Your skin should be clean and dry, with no oils or lotions. You should not be wearing a bra or underwire because the wire can interfere with the ECG.

An ECG is done by attaching electrodes to your chest, arms or legs and using sticky gel to record the electrical signals of your heart. This test is used to diagnose certain heart diseases and monitor the function of artificial cardiac pacemakers.

A typical ECG tracing shows several different waves: the P wave in the atria, the QRS complex in the ventricles and the T wave in the atria and ventricles. It also sometimes shows a U wave, which is a Purkinje repolarization wave.

In addition, a heart rhythm called ventricular fibrillation can be seen when the normal waves of the ECG are not present, which means the heart is beating extremely quickly and irregularly and cannot pump blood properly. Ventricular fibrillation can cause sudden death if it is not treated.

Cardiac arrest can happen suddenly, but most people who have it survive if they get medical help fast. Your doctor will run tests to find out what caused the problem and what treatment you need to restore your heart's normal rhythm.

Your doctor will also give you medicines to keep your heart working normally and reduce your risk of sudden death. These drugs may include potassium, magnesium and other hormones. They may also contain chemicals that slow down the rate at which your heart can beat, or that can help to strengthen your heart's contractions.

The heart's electrical signals can be confused by other things in your body that are not working well, such as high blood pressure or diabetes. In this study, we developed a method that predicts whether a patient is likely to have an episode of cardiac arrest (PEA) in the coming 24 h. We compared the ECGs of patients who had PEA with ECGs of patients who did not have an episode.

ECG in Shock

Cardiac Shock is the leading cause of mortality after a heart attack and is more common in women and people with coronary artery disease. Patients can also develop CS if they have other conditions that decrease their ability to produce enough blood, such as a severe form of congestive heart failure or kidney disease.

Infections, heart valve damage, and ventricular dysfunction are other risk factors for CS. It is most common in patients with acute myocardial infarction, but it can happen in many other situations as well.

The electrocardiogram (ECG) is an important diagnostic test

for CS, but it can be difficult to identify the changes that occur during an episode of CS. These changes are sometimes nonspecific and not enough to diagnose a cardiac condition, but they can make the difference between life and death.

A number of morphological and electrical changes on the ECG can indicate a change in heart function, such as a sudden increase in cardiac output, a change in cardiac rhythm, or an interruption of cardiac conduction. These changes can be identified by an experienced examiner or a specialist in heart rhythm and electrocardiography, or they can be spotted by a trained layperson.

To measure the degree of change in cardiac output, your healthcare provider might order a catheterization procedure that uses a tube to inject a dye into a blood vessel. This dye shows the flow of blood to your heart and allows your doctor to see how much of each beat your heart is pumping out.

Your healthcare provider will also assess your vital signs, such as your heart rate and pulse pressure. These tests will tell your doctor how your heart is functioning and whether your organs are coping with the extra blood.

If the results of these tests show that your heart is not able to produce enough blood, your healthcare provider will use drugs and medical procedures to try to get more blood to your organs. These may include intravenous (IV) nitroprusside or a mechanical-assist device called an intra-aortic balloon pump.

The goal of treatment is to return the heart to a normal rhythm and raise your blood pressure. If these treatments do not work, your healthcare provider might need to perform other tests to determine the cause of your shock and the best course of treatment.

A specialized ECG score has been developed to evaluate the degree of change in cardiac output and can be used for quick diagnosis of CS. The score integrates different relevant factors of the ECG into a single index and can be used conveniently. It can be a reliable substitution for the LVEF or SI and can also be used to detect the onset of a haemodynamic derangement.

ECG in Acute Coronary Syndrome

The electrocardiogram (ECG) is one of the most accessible and commonly used diagnostic tools for patients arriving at an emergency department with acute chest pain suggestive of coronary artery disease. However, there is still considerable debate concerning the prognostic value of ECG findings in ACS and the relationship between ECG changes and clinical outcome.

ST-segment elevation versus ST-segment depression on the ECG in acute coronary syndrome

In patients with acute coronary syndrome, ST-segment elevation is considered to be the most predictive diagnostic marker for immediate intervention in the form of percutaneous coronary intervention (PCI) and/or thrombolysis. The presence of

ST-segment elevation on the ECG indicates severe ischemia, and therefore a higher risk of angiographic heart disease and an increased probability of early cardiovascular morbidity and mortality.

A subgroup of patients presenting with acute coronary syndrome in the GUSTO-IIb trial had a significantly higher rate of early invasive evaluation when they had ST-segment elevation on their ECG compared with the group without this finding. A multivariable model showed that this difference in initial treatment was due to the higher incidence of myocardial infarction among those with a ST-segment elevation on their admission ECG (hazard ratio, 1.08; 95% confidence interval, 0.88-1.26; P 0.0001). This difference was more prominent in patients with an earlier ST-segment elevation than in those with a later one (hazard ratio, 2.11; 95% confidence interval, 1.04-3.08; P 0.0001).

Dynamic ST-segment elevation and depression on the ECG in acute coronary artery disease

The dynamic nature of ACS means that some abnormalities may not be apparent until symptoms have started. A normal ECG recorded during an asymptomatic period, or when the patient is symptom-free, usually becomes abnormal when symptoms are present and may "pseudonormalize" over time, thus making the diagnosis of ACS even more challenging. The same pattern may be seen when an individual is tachycardic, as this could result in ST-segment depression in the precordial leads that are otherwise considered to be indicative of ischemia [3, 4].

Up-sloping ST-segment depression and positive T waves on the ECG are also common in patients with non-ST-segment elevation ACS (NSTE-ACS) who are tachycardic. Increasingly, this is seen in cases of subtotal occlusion with impaired flow in the coronary arteries [6, 18].

In the context of the GUSTO-IIb trial, the authors compared the predictive value of a number of ECG presentations for ACS with the ability to predict death or myocardial reinfarction during the first 30 days of follow-up. The authors found that a majority of ED physicians use symptoms as the most important diagnostic tool to grade their suspicion of ACS when considering their patients' ECGs. In the regression models comparing obvious/strong with vague/no suspicion of ACS, symptoms typical of ACS were considerably more often associated with a strong suspicion of ACS than an ischemic ECG or a pathological initial TnT. In addition, the occurrence of non-suspicious symptoms was significantly more frequent in those who had an obvious/strong suspicion of ACS than in those who had a vague/no suspicion.

Electrocardiogram (ECG) in Cardiogenic Shock

A standard electrocardiogram (ECG) is a test that checks your heart rhythm. Your doctor may order an ECG to look for heart problems, or to check your risk for developing one.

It's a serious medical emergency that can occur at any age, but is most common in people who have had a heart attack. It's usually treated with medications to lower blood pressure and correct the heart rhythm. In severe cases, doctors may use a special machine to pump your blood.

Signs and symptoms of cardiogenic shock include low urine production, cold arms and legs, altered level of consciousness and changes in your heart rate and blood pressure. You may also have other signs of heart failure, such as low oxygen levels in your blood.

You'll be asked to lie still for a few minutes while your heart rate is monitored by a machine. You'll have to be comfortable and not move or talk while you're lying down, because this can interfere with the results.

Your ECG might reveal an ST-segment deviation, which is a sign that your heart's electrical system is not working correctly. This can indicate an irregular heart rhythm, which is a major cause of death in people with coronary artery disease.

ACS patients have a higher risk of developing cardiogenic shock than other people. It's especially dangerous if you've had a heart attack, or if you have a condition like hypertension.

Researchers are trying to find ways to treat it more quickly. There's no cure for it yet, but the early detection and treatment of CS can decrease your risk for death.

In some countries, doctors have a special type of ECG called a pulse oximeter that can detect a sudden change in heart rate or blood pressure. It's not as accurate as a standard ECG, but it can tell your doctor whether you're having a heart attack or have other serious conditions.

A doctor might also recommend a Holter monitor, which records your ECG for several hours or days at a time. A holder monitor can be a good choice if you have a family history of heart disease.

In a new study, researchers found that ECG scores were more accurate at predicting mortality in patients with cardiogenic shock than LVEF or SI. It was also better at identifying patients with the condition who needed urgent treatment, including surgery or other procedures to improve blood flow to the heart.

Chapter 8.
ECG Artifacts

Electrocardiograph (ECG) artifacts are a class of distortions in the electrocardiogram, not related to cardiac electrical activity. They can affect the quality of an ECG and are usually easy to miss as they may not resemble any specific pattern, and may not be accompanied by other diagnostic changes that may mimic a genuine abnormality.

The most common ECG artifacts are motion artifacts and electrical interference from a nearby electronic device. Examples of these include a 100 Hz background distorted signal from fluorescent lights, or a stray ECG signal that can be detected by a well-designed EKG machine (see Table 4.5 on page 58).

There are many types of movement related artifacts including tremor, shivering, fever induced shaking and muscle twitching. Often these may occur as a result of the patient moving his limbs, or as a result of a simple movement such as brushing his hair.

Other types of ECG artifacts are a little more difficult to identify and explain. These may be due to a lack of proper grounding of the ECG machine, a poorly placed lead on the body, or incorrect placement of leads and cables.

The best way to avoid these common pitfalls is to be aware of them and keep a high degree of vigilance in the event that one does occur. This will help you to quickly and effectively assess the possible causes of the aforementioned cardio graphic changes, and will prevent unnecessary testing and therapeutic interventions for your patient.

An Overview of ECG Artifacts

ECG artifacts are alterations in the electrocardiogram that are not related to cardiac electrical activity and can lead to the distortion of normal components of the ECG. They are commonly a cause for misdiagnosis and unnecessary testing or treatments. This article will present two cases and explore some of the internal and external causes of ECG artifacts.

Motion artifacts are produced by the patient's movements (tremors and shivering). They can also be caused by nearby electrical interference. For example, a fluorescent lamp can distort the baseline by 100 Hz causing a squiggly or irregular waveform, which may be mistaken for atrial fibrillation.

Movement disorders, such as Parkinson's disease, can produce a tremor with no apparent cause and may result in the occurrence of baseline wander artifact. These are often easily overlooked and may be confused with atrial flutter or fibrillation.

Electrode misplacement can cause the onset of ECG artifacts, including resembling atrial fibrillation and tall T waves. Early identification and replacement of electrodes can save unnecessary testing and treatment.

Common ECG artifacts include:

Electrical noise from mains wiring can cause a wavy line or straight line on the ECG trace that is reminiscent of systole and atrial flutter. This can occur when the lead wires are incorrectly placed or if the machine is not properly plugged in.

Improper electrode placement can also lead to the onset of ECG artifacts, as can the wrong type of leads being used. These can resemble a heart block or the onset of a life-threatening arrhythmia.

Artifacts can also be caused by poor signal quality. This can be a problem when recording ECGs in busy primary care practices as thousands of 12 lead ECGs are performed daily and the results can be inaccurate.

These problems can be avoided by using fresh and high-quality electrodes, making sure the wires are fully inserted into the machine and that the lead cables are not accidentally plugged in. The ECG can also be prevented from being distorted by keeping the electrode skin interface stable.

Electrode and lead placement can also be a cause of ECG artifacts, particularly in patients with a history of heart attack or an existing arrhythmia. It can be difficult to spot this artifact, so it is essential that the GP takes extra care with electrode placement.

Other common sources of ECG artifacts are external and internal interference from equipment within the room, such as cell phones and medical devices. These interferences can make the ECG trace appear distorted and can be easily reduced by abrading the patient's skin.

Interference can also be prevented by monitoring a range of settings on the monitor, such as the power frequency, filtering and alarm sensitivity. For example, a higher power filter setting can reduce the likelihood of displaying the artifact and improve trace quality.

Several methods have been developed to remove these unwanted ECG artifacts, including template subtraction and adaptive filters. However, these methods require reference signals or the original sEMG to be filtered. The present study aims to develop a new method that can eliminate the artifacts from single-channel sEMG recordings. This method uses fully convolutional neural networks to achieve this goal and is able to reduce the number of references needed to eliminate the artifacts.

Types of ECG Artifacts

There are many different types of ECG artifacts, which may be caused by a variety of factors. These include tremor, movement, and electrical interference. These should not be confused with a real abnormality in the ECG such as atrial fibrillation, which can have a different appearance in an ECG.

Electrode misplacements: Loose wires, wavy lines, and tall T waves can produce ECG artifacts that mimic a wide complex of ventricular tachycardia or a premature contraction (STE). Early identification and replacement of electrodes can prevent unnecessary therapy.

Motion artifacts: these are generated by a patient shaking with rhythmic movements and can be related to Parkinson's disease, cerebellar tremor, anxiety, hyperthyroidism, multiple sclerosis, or drugs such as amphetamines and benzodiazepines.

These artifacts may be difficult to eliminate, especially when they are in the spectral band below 100 Hz. They can be removed using template subtraction or adaptive filtering, both of which are based on the principle of estimating the fluctuation around linear trend in the monopolar channel.

The accuracy of the methods varies depending on the number of coarse artifacts and the signal amplitude. We used a range of values, and 90% to 97% of the useful signal parts were preserved in cECG recordings with at least one coarse artifact.

We also tested the performance of the method on cECG recordings that had been subjected to various amounts of stimulation by driving or lying on a bed. In both cases, the method was able to eliminate artifacts by a significant amount of time.

Reducing cECG Artifacts: Coarse artifacts in cECG recordings are a common problem and can make it difficult to analyze a cECG. These artifacts can have a high amplitude and can cause a change in the signal spectral properties, which can make it hard to interpret the cECG.

This can result in problems with classification of cECG signals or their analysis by cardiovascular parameters. The removal of coarse artifacts from cECG signals may increase their reliability and accuracy for classification purposes.

However, the extraction of spikes from cECG is not an easy task because the cECG signal recorded by the electrodes is very noisy and consists of numerous peaks. In this context, we developed a robust ECG spike extraction algorithm, which can be applied to the monopolar channel and to the ECG signals of moving subjects.

In this study, we analyzed the accuracy of the proposed method on the cECG recordings of patients while lying on a bed and driving in the city and on the open road. We compared the results of the method with the opinions of experts.

The method was successful in reducing cECG artifacts, with a higher percentage of the signal being preserved than that observed by the experts. The method was able to significantly eliminate cECG artifacts during both driving and sleeping in bed, resulting in improved cECG signal quality. The method is safe to use, has a small memory footprint, and can be implemented quickly and efficiently.

Causes of ECG Artifacts

Electrocardiogram (ECG) artifacts are disturbances in the signal that may alter its amplitude, frequency and morphology. These can be caused by a variety of factors, both internal and external, which can mask the underlying cause of a patient's abnormalities and prevent an accurate diagnosis. Incorrectly interpreted ECGs can lead to unnecessary tests and interventions, such as anticoagulation in the case of ischemia or resuscitation in the case of heart arrhythmia.

Non-physiological sources of ECG artifacts include 60 hertz mains noise, electromagnetic induction, electrode movement and static electricity. In addition, other equipment such as a computer or telephone in the room can generate a similar disturbance on the ECG.

Static electricity: this is the most common cause of ECG artifacts and can be caused by many different things including broken wiring, poor connections between cables and electrodes and accumulated static electricity in the device. This can be a major source of distorted ECGs and must be prevented by proper quality control measures.

Infection and other medical conditions can also result in ECG artifacts as these may cause a reduction in the sensitivity of the device to detect electrical activity. Therefore, it is important to ensure the device is disinfected regularly and that all leads are well positioned in the body.

Other causes of ECG artifacts include skin impedance and muscle movement. The skin's resistance to the flow of electricity through it can impede the transmission of electrical signals from the heart, to the sensor element in the electrode. This can be avoided by using fresh, high-quality electrodes and by ensuring that the cabling is properly connected to the monitor.

Motion: During normal walking, patients can produce movement artifacts on the ECG trace due to their large swings of muscles. Tremors and shivering also can generate movement artifacts on the ECG.

ECG tracings can also be affected by the presence of other devices such as power cords, infusion pumps, ventilators and in some cases, the ECG monitor itself. Taking the time to look at a patient's tracing and check for any 'non-conventional' tracing patterns can help to identify these traces as they may indicate the presence of other disorders or conditions.

Unwanted ECG artifacts can be prevented by identifying and removing all the devices that can interfere with the trace. This will not only improve the trace quality but will also prevent unwanted alarms from being triggered.

Changing the way, you view and interpret ECGs will also help to avoid c. Causes of ECG artifacts in the future.

Having the knowledge of the various sources of ECG artifacts can save you time and money in the long run. By identifying these problems early, you can avoid misdiagnosis and unnecessary testing or intervention. Having the right training and tools will also ensure you are able to make the correct diagnosis in all situations.

ECG Artifact Recognition

Artifacts are alterations in the ECG waveform that are not caused by electrical activity of the heart. Several factors can cause these alterations. These include external and internal interference, tremors and movement disorders. Moreover, ECG artifacts can also be due to medical devices.

ECG signal quality is a critical issue in clinical applications as it can help in diagnosing an abnormality of the heart. A poor signal can lead to misdiagnosis, unnecessary tests and treatments or even death. It is important to detect these artifacts and remove them to ensure that the patients' electrocardiogram (ECG) reading is accurate and does not pose any risk to their life.

The quality of the ECG can be assessed by analyzing signal metrics such as flatness, impulses and Gaussian noise within the ECG signal. This can be accomplished by using algorithms that can detect such features. However, it is a challenging task to develop such algorithms as they may affect the signal's legibility and require the entire unmodified waveform for analysis.

Various sources of electrical artifacts on the ECG can occur due to line current, muscle tremors or hiccups, resuscitation, deep brain stimulation, cardiopulmonary resuscitation (CPR), electrolyte imbalance, wrong placement of an electrode and patient's body temperature. Some of these artifacts, such as the left arm lead reversal can be easily mistaken for atrial fibrillation.

In the present study, we examined the feasibility of removing motion artifacts from sensing-enabled neurostimulators. We used a simultaneous monopolar montage as a reference to obtain distinct R-waves in the bipolar LFP recordings and filtered the signals to remove the artifacts by using existing methods such as template subtraction and adaptive filtering.

We evaluated the performance of these methods in a simulation environment. The resulting signal quality metrics, such as the ratio of peak-to-sinusoidal-peak squared length error (RMSLE) and the average signal-to-noise-ratio (ASN), are used to evaluate the effectiveness of the ECG artifact removal algorithms. The results showed that both template subtraction and adaptive filtering removed the motion artifacts in the contaminated LFPs without any additional filtering of DBS artifacts, which were not significantly influenced by the magnitude of the residual DBS artifacts.

In the future, it is essential to improve the effectiveness of these methods and to develop algorithms that can perform ECG artifact removal in real time. The use of these algorithms could help physicians and nurses to quickly diagnose an abnormality of the heart. They could also help in identifying potential causes of a patient's deteriorating condition and assist in determining the correct course of action.

Chapter 9.
ECG Interpretation

A good ECG requires more than just a cursory glance, it requires a well-designed study plan that incorporates all the critical elements of the heart's operating system.

The best way to accomplish this is by reading a good ECG book, attending an effective classroom course and practicing with real-life ECGs - all while observing patients in the midst of their cardiac emergencies. The result is a solid foundation on which to build your clinical skills and a competitive edge on your peers.

What are the most important elements to consider when interpreting an ECG?

One of the most critical aspects is understanding what each electrode represents on the ECG and how they interact with each other.

This will ensure that you are able to pick out the most vital information to make your patient care decisions in the least amount of time and with the most accuracy.

There are a multitude of ECG books and resources available to help you with this task. The best resource is the one that best suits your needs and educational objectives. A good book will be able to show you the best ways to learn this crucial skill, and how to implement this knowledge to improve patient care and your career. The art of interpretation will become second nature to you as you become more confident in putting your brain and heart to work.

Reflection on the Importance of ECG Interpretation in Healthcare

ECGs are important for diagnosing cardiovascular diseases, such as heart attacks or high blood pressure. They can also be used to assess artificial cardiac pacemakers or monitor the effects of medications on your heart. They are a relatively low-cost test and are painless to perform.

Misinterpretation of the ECG is a major concern because it can lead to wrong diagnosis and delay appropriate treatment, which in turn leads to poor patient outcomes. Although physicians can learn to interpret ECGs, the skill is not easy to develop and requires continuous practice. There is an urgent need for improved educational methods, as well as increased recognition and respect for the importance of this skill.

Training in ECG interpretation has been criticized for its lack of focus across medical training programs. This has led to a loss of competency in the skill and increased reliance on computer-based ECG analysis for aiding in clinical decision making.

A large number of studies have shown that ECG interpretation skills are a significant factor in a physician's ability to diagnose and treat patients, and that misinterpretation can have adverse consequences. Nevertheless, there is little evidence about the optimal methods for teaching, assessing, and maintaining this skill.

The current review was designed to systematically identify and summarize published research that measured the accuracy of physicians' ECG interpretations. We focused on studies that assessed interpretation accuracy in a controlled (educational) test setting, which permits adjudication relative to a single correct response.

Our analysis identified 78 studies that assessed the accuracy of physicians' ECG interpretations. The average accuracy score was 54% (interquartile range, 44% to 65%). These findings are consistent with other studies that have reported low accuracy.

Accuracy scores were higher with more training and specialization (medical students, residents, physicians in no cardiology practice, and cardiologists), but still varied widely. These results suggest that physicians at all training levels were disadvantaged in ECG interpretation, even after educational interventions.

Presentation of clinical history on ECGs impacts visual appraisal and ECG interpretation

Healthcare-practitioners skilled in 12-lead ECG interpretation were asked to counterbalance viewing nine different ECGs in arbitrary sequence with or without a brief history of the presenting complaint. A Hellinger-distance calculation was used to determine eye-movement transitions at two granularity levels: between the ECG leads, and between smaller grid-cells.

We found that a longer patient history significantly affects the visual appraisal of a 12-lead ECG and subsequently, the interpretation of this ECG. The effect of a history is likely to be greater for complex ECGs, but may have an impact on simpler ones as well.

ECG interpretation is an essential skill for most physicians. Therefore, improving ECG education and assessment is an essential component for achieving the highest quality of care. To this end, standardized competencies, educational resources, and mastery benchmarks should be developed. The goal is to re-educate physicians and trainees in the art of accurate ECG interpretation, thereby enabling them to detect and diagnose cardiovascular disease with confidence and competence.

Conclusion

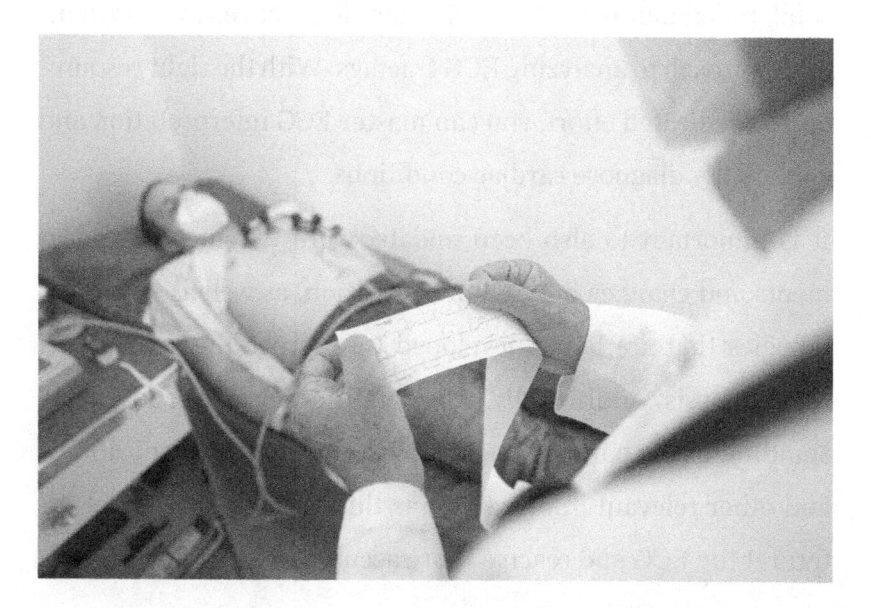

Interpreting an ECG (electrocardiogram) requires a strong understanding of the electrical signals generated by the heart and how they are recorded on the ECG paper. As a beginner, it is important to first familiarize yourself with the different waves and intervals present on an ECG tracing and understand their significance in evaluating heart function.

In order to pass an exam on ECG interpretation, you should focus on practicing with different ECG tracings and understanding the changes in waveform and intervals that occur in different cardiac conditions. Additionally, it is important to understand the use of ECG in diagnosing various cardiac conditions such as arrhythmias, myocardial infarction, and electrolyte imbalances, among others.

To summarize, passing an ECG interpretation exam requires a solid understanding of the basics, ample practice, and a systematic approach to analyzing ECG tracings. With the right resources and dedicated effort, you can master ECG interpretation and confidently diagnose cardiac conditions.

It is important to also keep updated with the latest advancements and changes in ECG interpretation, as well as new technologies that are being developed to improve the accuracy of ECG analysis. Additionally, it is helpful to have a good understanding of the patient's medical history, current medications, and other relevant information, as this can help you better interpret the ECG and reach a more accurate diagnosis.

Furthermore, it is essential to communicate your findings and recommendations effectively to other healthcare providers, as ECG interpretation forms an integral part of patient care. In addition, you should be aware of the limitations of ECG interpretation, as well as the importance of obtaining additional tests, such as echocardiograms or cardiac catheterizations, to confirm your diagnoses.

In conclusion, ECG interpretation is a complex and ever-evolving field, but with dedication and a strong foundation of knowledge, you can become an expert in this area and make a valuable contribution to patient care.

Made in United States
North Haven, CT
29 September 2023